O P M

OXFORD PAIN MANAGEMENT LIBRARY

Trigeminal Neuralgia and Other Cranial Neuralgias

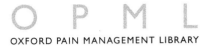

OXFORD PAIN MANAGEMENT LIBRARY

Trigeminal Neuralgia and Other Cranial Neuralgias

A Practical Personalized Holistic Approach

Edited by

Joanna M. Zakrzewska

Hon. Professor of Pain in Relation to Oral Medicine, University College London
Consultant University College Hospitals NHS Foundation Trust, London, UK

Turo Nurmikko

Hon. Professor, The Walton Centre NHS Foundation Trust, Liverpool, UK

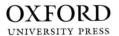

OXFORD
UNIVERSITY PRESS

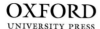

UNIVERSITY PRESS

Great Clarendon Street, Oxford, OX2 6DP,
United Kingdom

Oxford University Press is a department of the University of Oxford.
It furthers the University's objective of excellence in research, scholarship,
and education by publishing worldwide. Oxford is a registered trade mark of
Oxford University Press in the UK and in certain other countries

Published in the United States of America by Oxford University Press
198 Madison Avenue, New York, NY 10016, United States of America

British Library Cataloguing in Publication Data

Data available

Library of Congress Control Number: 2021947341

ISBN 978–0–19–887160–6

DOI: 10.1093/med/9780198871606.001.0001

Printed and bound by
CPI Group (UK) Ltd, Croydon, CR0 4YY

Oxford University Press makes no representation, express or implied, that the
drug dosages in this book are correct. Readers must therefore always check
the product information and clinical procedures with the most up-to-date
published product information and data sheets provided by the manufacturers
and the most recent codes of conduct and safety regulations. The authors and
the publishers do not accept responsibility or legal liability for any errors in the
text or for the misuse or misapplication of material in this work. Except where
otherwise stated, drug dosages and recommendations are for the non-pregnant
adult who is not breast-feeding

Links to third party websites are provided by Oxford in good faith and
for information only. Oxford disclaims any responsibility for the materials
contained in any third party website referenced in this work.

Foreword

Orofacial pain affects up to 10% of the adult population. The suffering of the individuals afflicted, and the extensive costs associated with both management and consequences, such as lost productivity, impaired physiological and psychological functioning, and low quality of life, are enormous problems for the individual and society. Before we had carbamazepine, that is, before we could treat patients with a dreadful disease such as trigeminal neuralgia, affected patients may have died—not from suicide as one would assume given the extreme shock-like pain, but from dehydration and starving—since these pain attacks are triggered by touching the face, chewing, or swallowing. To the present day, trigeminal neuralgia is a case of emergency.

Knowing this, it is mind-boggling how little money is spent to better understand and consequently treat chronic facial pain syndromes. Even worse, medical students in some countries learn little about facial pain syndromes. Indeed, if not trained as a neurologist or neurosurgeon, they usually have few chances during the long journey to become a medical doctor to be in contact with these patients and put this diagnosis into perspective when considering all other facial pain, and also headache syndromes. Although trigeminal neuralgia is literally a spot diagnosis, it is still under- and overdiagnosed in the clinical setting, since many patients who should have been given the diagnosis do not get it (and are consequently not treated correctly); there are also patients who have been diagnosed with trigeminal neuralgia but in fact suffer from another type of facial pain or headache. Furthermore, if the classic medication carbamazepine is not effective or otherwise not well tolerated, most clinicians are at a loss of what to do next. Meanwhile, the classification is refined, new medications are tested, and the scientific efforts to better understand the pathophysiological background increase, with the consequence of a wealth of new information every year.

There is, therefore, a clear need to get a better grasp on an ever-evolving field of what is a seemingly straightforward diagnosis. This handbook serves exactly this need not just for clinicians but also for clinical scientists: it is comprehensive, timely, and an easy read. Readers will be rewarded with a complete and current overview of the field, emphasizing the connection between pathophysiological background and practical therapeutic applications in medicine. Other cranial neuralgias and the diagnostic pitfalls of painful trigeminal neuropathy are contrasted and the classic differential diagnosis of short-lasting unilateral neuralgiform headache attack (SUNHA) and other short-lived trigeminal autonomic headaches are expertly described. The handbook is divided into 19 sections that provide a thoroughly updated resource that will increase the knowledge of the various forms of facial pain as well as the contribution of biological sciences for the understanding of the pathophysiology. It provides clear evidence-based pointers for pharmacological and also surgical treatments. The broad range of different skills and backgrounds of the editors and contributing authors of this book not only provide a guarantee of its undisputed scientific quality, but also give it an international dimension.

Books have been written about trigeminal neuralgia. However, the present handbook brings an important perspective to this problem, that is, it underlines the importance of the biopsychosocial model for patient encounters. Indeed, patients and patient support groups alike will have their say, and I urge you to have a look at Chapter 19 on the 'face2face' project. This patient-to-clinician interaction is not often seen in neurology or neurosurgery dealing with trigeminal neuralgia where it is only too often that the patient is reduced to a mechanistic vessel–nerve contact. I enjoyed reading this book. It should get the recognition it deserves being that it is a comprehensive pain syndrome reference source for whoever opens it.

Arne May

Preface

Welcome to a novel book on trigeminal neuralgia and other cranial neuralgias.
Why this book now? In the last few years, there has been a growing interest in cranial neuralgias and related conditions. It has been driven by advances in pathophysiology, neuropharmacology, neurophysiology, neuroimaging, interventional techniques, and social sciences and resulted in a major shift in the way we are thinking about and dealing with these painful conditions. Guidelines are increasingly evidence based and clinical practice is following the trend. International disease classification systems, such as the ICHD-3 and ICOP, joint ventures between the International Headache Society and International Association for the Study of Pain, published in 2018 and 2020, and the ICD-11 by the World Health Organization in 2020, rely more than earlier editions on aetiology, phenotyping, and genotyping as their bases of nosology and taxonomy of cranial neuralgias. There is an increasing demand for precision diagnosis to ensure clinicians deliver optimal treatment. To deliver best treatment we need to provide personalized care which involves shared decision-making. Systematic reviews have shown that both healthcare professionals and patients overestimate the effects of treatment and underestimate harm. An initiative in the UK, Rethinking Medicine (https://rethinkingmedicine.org.uk/) suggests that we need to focus more on quality of life and well-being in order to improve healthcare. Pain medicine has long recognized the psychosocial consequences of pain and its impact on patients' quality of life. The biopsychosocial approach to pain management using a multidisciplinary team is similarly well established and is essential in the cranial neuralgias. Clinical research has revealed promising vistas across the field, ranging from genomics to applied neuroimaging and development of new drugs. This book represents an endeavour to bring together all the newest developments in the field in a format that offers guidance on all aspects of clinical practice.

The reader will be able to familiarize themselves with the joint efforts of a distinguished international group of experts from a wide range of specialities who have given much of their time to prepare their contributions in the style we asked for. Our aim has been to present what is important in the successful clinical management of a patient with any given cranial neuralgia in a concise, yet comprehensive fashion. Patient experience has been given a prominent platform. Their narratives are reflected in patient advocacy group presentations and through visual arts.

This book aims to maximize the learning experience and its effectiveness, using a variety of methods. It is a recognition of the fact that we all have different learning styles—here, we are trying to accommodate them. There are mind maps and algorithms for those who learn best through visual material. Others may like to be introduced to a topic with a patient scenario, so these are presented in each topic (each representing a real patient). Some may wish to see the key points to remind themselves whether they are on the right path, whereas others may want more in-depth evidence to support management. The reader has an opportunity to test their skills at the end of each chapter with the answers being provided at the end of the book. For patients who seek reliable information on their pain, there is a lay summary at the end of each chapter. We have resisted the urge to include vast numbers of references and instead provide key recommended texts, with online links to in-depth material for those who want to explore a given topic beyond the scope of this book. The introduction chapter contains some of the key references which are common to many of the chapters.

We hope this book will guide you, dear reader, through the diagnostic maze of conditions leading to facial pain—with an emphasis on the cranial neuralgias usually discussed superficially in pain textbooks.

This book would not have been possible without the generous time our experts round the world have given to ensure we are bringing you the very latest high-quality information. We are very grateful for their contributions and cooperation in helping us keep to a consistent style. We would like to thank Adrian Hale, a trigeminal neuralgia patient, who prepared several graphics for the book. Oxford University Press have been very encouraging and supportive in putting together this handbook. Joanna received some funding from the Department of Health's National Institute for Health Research Biomedical Research Centre at University College London Hospitals NHS Foundation Trust and University College London (UCLH/UCL) and support from the Facial Pain Unit and Pain Management Centre at UCLH. We are both grateful to our spouses who put up with the hours we spent putting this volume together and enabled us to work as a productive team. Perhaps the COVID-19 pandemic helped us put this together in a relatively short space of time due to a reduction in our usual conferences round the world and deployments from our usual work. Thank you to everyone who will spread the word about this group of conditions and help patients live well with their pain.

Contents

Contributors

Jillie Abbott
Former
Chair & Trustee of the Trigeminal
   Neuralgia Association UK
Copthorne
West Sussex, UK

**Vishal R. Aggarwal,
BDS, MFDSRCS, MPH, PhD,
FCGDent**
Clinical Associate Professor
School of Dentistry
University of Leeds
Leeds, UK

Mohammed A. Amer, MD
Intern Physician
Shmaisani Hospital
Department of Clinical Education
   School of Medicine
University of Jordan
Amman, Jordan

**Lene Baad-Hansen, DDS, PhD,
Dr. Odont.**
Professor and Deputy Head for
   Research
Department of Dentistry and
   Oral Health
Aarhus University
Aarhus, Denmark

Anish Bahra, FRCP, MD
Consultant Neurologist
Neurology and Headache Service
Barts Health and the National Hospital
   for Neurology and Neurosurgery
London, UK

Kim J. Burchiel, MD, FACS
Professor
Department of Neurological Surgery
Oregon Health and Science University
Portland, OR, USA

William P. Cheshire Jr, MD
Professor
Department of Neurology
Mayo Clinic
Jacksonville, FL, USA

**H. Clare Daniel, DClinPsych,
BSc (Hons), MBA**
Chief Psychologist
Buckinghamshire Healthcare Trust
Buckinghamshire, UK

Karen D. Davis, PhD
Professor
Department of Surgery and Institute of
   Medical Science
University of Toronto
Senior Scientist and Head,
   Division of Brain
Imaging and Behaviour Krembil Brain
   Institute, Krembil Research Institute
University Health Network
Toronto, ON, Canada

Gianfranco De Stefano, MD
Department of Human Neurosciences
Sapienza University
Rome, Italy

Giulia Di Stefano, MD, PhD
Researcher
Department of Human Neuroscience
Sapienza University
Rome, Italy

Scott R. Diehl, BS, PhD
Professor
Department of Oral Biology
Rutgers School of Dental Medicine
   Rutgers
Newark, NJ, USA

Ann Eastman
Retired Graphic Designer

Matteo Fuccaro, MD
Cinical Fellow
Headache and Facial Pain Service
Guy's and St Thomas' NHS
  Foundation Trust
London, UK

Alison Glenn
Former Trigeminal Neuralgia Patient
Huntingdon, Cambridgeshire

**Mojgan Hodaie, MD,
MSc, FRCSC**
Professor
Department of Surgery
University of Toronto
Toronto, ON, Canada

Satu K. Jääskeläinen, MD, PhD
Professor
Department of Clinical Neurophysiology
Turku University Hospital, University
  of Turku
Turku, Finland

Giorgio Lambru, PhD
Consultant Neurologist and Honorary
  Senior Lecturer
Headache Centre, Medical Specialities,
Guy's and St Thomas' NHS Foundation
  Trust and Kings' College London
London, UK

Stine Maarbjerg, MD, PhD
Medical Doctor and Post Doc
Department of Neurology, Danish
  Headache Center
Rigshospitalet—Glostrup
Glostrup, Denmark

**Imran Noorani, MB Chir,
MRCS, PhD**
Clinical Lecturer in Neurosurgery
Department of Neurosurgery
University College London
London, UK

Turo Nurmikko, MD, PhD
Hon. Professor, The Walton Centre
  NHS Foundation Trust
Pain Relief Foundation Chair of Pain
  Science (ret.)
University of Liverpool
Liverpool, UK

**Francis O'Neill, PhD, MBChB,
FDSRCPS**
Senior Lecturer/Consultant in Oral
  Surgery
Dental School
University of Liverpool
Liverpool, UK

Mark Obermann, MD
Head of Department, Associate
  Professor
Department of Neurology
Hospital Weser-Egge, and University of
  Duisburg-Essen
Hoexter, Germany

Deborah Padfield, PhD
Senior Lecturer in Arts & Health
  Humanities
Institute of Medical and Biomedical
  Education
St George's, University of London
Lecturer Slade School of Fine
  Art, University College London
Gower Street
London, UK

Claire Patterson
Trigeminal Neuralgia Patient
Founder/CEO
NA
Trigeminal Neuralgia Association—USA
Gainesville, FL, USA

Jean Régis, MD
Chief of Service
Department of Neurosurgeon
Aix Marseille University Functional
  Neurosurgery Service & Radiosurgery
CHU Timone, Marseille, France

Raymond F. Sekula Jr, MD, MBA
Professor of Neurological Surgery
Columbia University Vagelos College of
 Physicians and Surgeons
NY, USA

Ze'ev Seltzer, DMD
Professor (Emeritus)
University of Toronto Faculties of
 Dentistry and Medicine
Oronto, ON, Canada

Elena Semino, MA, PhD
Professor and Director of ESRC Centre
 for Corpus Approaches to Social
 Science
Department of Linguistics and English
 Language
Lancaster University, UK

Marc Sindou, MD, DSc, DHC
Professor Emeritus Neurosurgery
Department of Neurosurgery
University of Lyon
Lyon, France

Claudia Sommer, MD
Professor
Department of Neurology
University of Würzburg
Würzburg, Germany

**Owen Sparrow, MMed, FRCS,
FRCSEd, FCS(SA)**
(Retired) Consultant Neurosurgeon
Department of Neurosurgery, Wessex
 Neurological Centre
University Hospital Southampton
Southampton, UK

**Pankaj Taneja, BDS, MJDF RCS
(Eng), MOralSurg, PG Cert, PhD**
Assistant Professor
Section of Oral and Maxillofacial Surgery
 and Oral Pathology, Department of
 Dentistry and Oral Health
Aarhus University
Aarhus, Denmark

**Pravin Thomas, MBBS, MD,
DNB, PGDCN, DEBN**
Consultant & Clinical Lead
Headache & Interventional Headache
 Neurology Services
NH Health City
Bangalore, India

Andrea Truini, MD, PhD
Professor of Neurology
Department of Human Neuroscience
Sapienza University
Rome, Italy

Constantin Tuleasca, MD, PhD
Neurosurgeon
Neurosurgery Service and Gamma
 Knife Center
Lausanne University Hospital (CHUV)
 and University of Lausanne (UNIL)
Lausanne, Switzerland

**Joanna M. Zakrzewska, BDS,
MBBChir, MD, FDSRCS,
FFDRCSI, FFPMRCA, FHEA**
Consultant/Hon Professor Oral
 Medicine
Royal National ENT & Eastman Dental
 Hospitals, and Pain Management
Centre NHNN, UCLH NHS
Foundation Trust, UCL
London, UK

Introduction

Joanna M. Zakrzewska and Turo Nurmikko

This book consists of 19 chapters, written by 37 authors from nine countries. We begin with a historical review of trigeminal neuralgia (TN) and related conditions in Chapter 2 which highlights the incredible range of treatments that have been used over the centuries. Over the years, understanding of the anatomy, physiology, and genetics of TN and, to a lesser extent, other conditions has advanced considerably although it still remains incomplete; this topic is covered in Chapter 3. Improved epidemiological statistics has helped to answer the question of how common these conditions are in Chapter 4.

Chapter 5 provides a detailed account of the diagnosis and assessment of facial pain. As we still do not have biomarkers for most pain conditions, it remains the remit of skilled clinicians to take a meticulous history which includes an assessment of psychological and social impacts of this condition. There have been considerable recent advances in our ability to image the nerves supplying the cranium while neurophysiological testing has shown utility in distinguishing different TN variants. Both methods are used to categorize patients for research and treatment purposes.

Changes to the classification of TN and other cranial neuralgias have been put forward by the International Headache Society (IHS), International Association for the Study of Pain (IASP), and World Health Organization (WHO) and are found in their respective classifications (ICHD-3, ICOP, and ICD-11). The nosology and symptomatology of TN are discussed in Chapters 6, 7, and 8 with a strong emphasis on differential diagnostics.

Pharmacological and surgical management of TN is covered by a range of experts in Chapters 9 and 10. They provide on the one hand a critical assessment of what is established and what is still compromised by uncertainties and controversies, and on the other hand offer practical guidance on individualized decision-making and patient management.

Chapter 11 is dedicated to painful trigeminal neuropathy, arguably the most important differential diagnosis of TN and a cause of much mismanagement of the latter. The following chapters, Chapters 12 and 13, deal with the clinical features and management of rare cranial neuralgias. Chapter 14 covers the four conditions classified by the IHS as the trigemino-autonomic cephalalgias. There are a range of common non-neuropathic facial pain conditions that often need to be excluded or included as a secondary diagnosis when managing patients with TN. These are covered briefly in Chapter 15.

Trigeminal and other cranial neuralgias have traditionally been managed as biomedical conditions and yet the impact of pain on quality of life and mood is significant. Suicide risk is higher than in the general population in patients with TN and cluster headaches. These factors need to be addressed in order to provide a holistic approach to the patient and to prevent suicides, and they are discussed in Chapter 16. Further support can be provided by patient support groups. The individual experiences of patients with TN are reflected in the material submitted to a patient-run forum and an analysis by a linguist has led to some fascinating conclusions which are discussed in Chapter 17.

As you go through the book, you will no doubt have numerous questions which we cannot answer, and we have summarized in Chapter 18 the challenges we face with cranial neuralgias but also the opportunities which potentially open up. We highlight issues that require more research and stress the need for international collaboration in order to provide improved care for our patients.

The final chapter, Chapter 19, provides images from a project used to visualize pain through photography. Patients with TN chartered their progress through their management by co-creating images with a visual artist. We hope they offer hope to all our patients that even if all pain cannot be eliminated, it is possible to

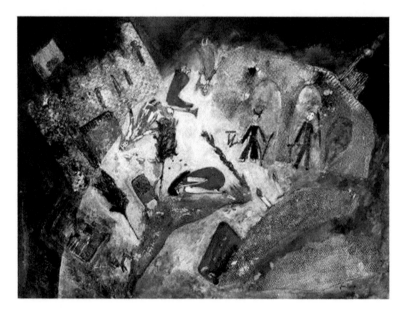

Figure 1.1 A day in my life
© Rosa Sepple.

CHAPTER 1

live well with pain. To many professionals, the non-verbal mediation of patient experience will be a vivid reminder of their struggle that doesn't always come through inside the sterile walls of a clinic.

Enjoy and learn so you can help Rosa (fig. 1.1) get off her island of isolation and pain and return to everyday life.

RECOMMENDED READING

The following are texts that are referred to in many of the chapters or are overall reviews:

Bendtsen L, Zakrzewska JM, Abbott J, et al. European Academy of Neurology guideline on trigeminal neuralgia. Eur J Neurol. 2019;26:831–49. doi: 10.1111/ene.13950

Bendtsen L, Zakrzewska JM, Heinskou TB, et al. Advances in diagnosis, classification, pathophysiology, and management of trigeminal neuralgia. Lancet Neurol. 2020;19:784–96. doi: 10.1016/S1474-4422(20)30233-7

Cephalalgia. Special issue: facial pain. Cephalalgia. 2017;377:603–719.

Headache Classification Committee of the International Headache Society (IHS). The International Classification of Headache Disorders, 3rd edition. Cephalalgia. 2018;38:1–211. doi: 10.1177/0333102417738202

International Classification of Orofacial Pain, 1st edition (ICOP). Cephalalgia. 2020;40:129–221. doi: 10.1177/0333102419893823

O'Callaghan L, Floden L, Vinikoor-Imler L, et al. Burden of illness of trigeminal neuralgia among patients managed in a specialist center in England. J Headache Pain. 2020;21:130. doi: 10.1186/s10194-020-01198-z

McMillan R, Zakrzewska J, Bahra A, et al. Guidelines for the management of trigeminal neuralgia. Royal College of Surgeons Faculty of Dental Surgery. 2021 https://www.rcseng.ac.uk/dental-faculties/fds/publications-guidelines/clinical-guidelines/

CHAPTER 2

History and classification of trigeminal neuralgia and other cranial neuralgias

Joanna M. Zakrzewska

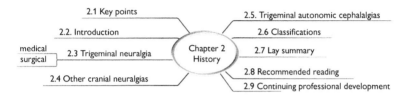

Figure 2.1 Plan of chapter

2.1 KEY POINTS

1. Trigeminal neuralgia was probably first described in the eleventh century but Andre and Fothergill first comprehensively described the features in the eighteenth century.
2. Bergouignan's report in 1942 on the use of phenytoin pioneered the use of antiepileptic drugs.
3. Although a wide variety of surgical techniques were being used from the eighteenth century onwards, it was the operating microscope that enabled microvascular decompression to become the surgical procedure of choice.
4. An internationally agreed classification system that includes trigeminal neuralgia and other craniofacial pain conditions has been developed.

2.2 Introduction

See Box 2.1.

> **Box 2.1** Scenario
>
> I am suffering,—and have suffered all night, and during the greater part of yesterday—insupportable torture from some complaint in the face—whether rheumatism, tic doloreux [sic] or what not, Heaven knows. I have had fomentations of various kinds, but with little or no relief, and am desperately beaten in consequence.
>
> Charles Dickens, letter, 2 October 1840
>
> I should have come to see you today, but I have been troubled with a raging face, and being out for a few minutes was visited by certain admonitory [warning] symptoms which sent me home again, faster than I came out.
>
> Charles Dickens, letter, 4 October 1840

2.3 Trigeminal neuralgia

It is postulated that trigeminal neuralgia (TN), also known as tic douloureux, was not known in ancient times as people did not live into old age. Aretaeus of Cappodocia and Avicenna, Arab physician (980–1037), are often credited with the first descriptions of TN but it is now suggested that they may have been describing facial spasm. Recent historical research suggests that Esmail Jorjani (1042–1137) in 'The Treasure of the Khwarazm Shah' gave an accurate description and even suggested that an artery was sitting on the nerve. In 1671, Fehr and Schmidt described symptoms in a German physician, Johannes Laurentius Bausch, who ultimately died of starvation due to pain which made it impossible to eat. Andre, in 1756, described tic douloureux as a painful twitch but the first comprehensive descriptions were by John Fothergill in a presentation he gave on 'of A painful affection of the face' at the Medical Society in London in 1773.

Looking at Table 2.1, we can see that Fothergill had provided many descriptions that are still valid today. Further features were gradually identified and by 1936 it was also recognized that there were 'atypical' presentations.

A very wide range of aetiological and pathophysiological causes have been put forward over the centuries.

2.3.1 Drug development

Over the centuries, a large number of drugs have been used (fig. 2.2) but it is postulated that Trousseau's (1877) name of 'névralgie epileptiform, tic consultif' for TN led Bergouignan in 1942 to use the antiepileptic phenytoin and in 1962, Blom published his trial of carbamazepine.

Table 2.1 Historical descriptions of trigeminal neuralgia

Trigeminal neuralgia	First descriptions, author, date
Location	Face and intraoral, Locke, 1677; maxillary area, Fehr and Schmidt, 1688
Unilateral	Avicenna; Jorjani, 1066; Massa, 1550; Andre, 1756
Trigeminal area	More right side, Tiffany, 1896; Harris, 1940; Adson, 1926
Divisions involved	Fehr and Schmidt, 1688; Tiffany, 1898; Moore, 1903; Adson, 1926; bilateral, Cushing, 1921
Character	Flash of fire, Locke, 1677; shooting, Patrick, 1914
Paroxysmal	Jorjani, 1066; Fothergill, 1783
Rapid onset and cessation	Locke, 1677; Fehr and Schmidt, 1688; Fothergill, 1783
Severity	Jorjani, 1066; varying, Locke, 1677; Fehr and Schmidt, 1688; Fothergill, 1783
Length of attacks	Intervals between attacks: 30 minutes, Locke, 1677; 15–30 seconds, Fothergill, 1783
Refractory period	Kugelberg Lindblom, 1959; Penman, 1968
Prodromal	Harris, 1909
Remission periods	Fehr and Schmidt, 1688; Fothergill, 1783; can be 6 months or longer, Rushton, 1957
Memorable onset	Harris, 1926; Penman, 1968
Light touch provoked	Chewing, swallowing, Massa, 1550; talking, touch, Locke, 1677; Andre, 1756; touch, Fothergill, 1783
Trigger areas	Patrick, 1914; Kugelberg and Lindblom, 1959; Henderson, 1967
Spasm of the face	Jorjani, 1066; Locke, 1677
After pain	Dull ache, Locke, 1677; continuous pain, Dandy, 1932; Henderson, 1967
Autonomic features	Eye watering, runny nose, Moore, 1903; lacrimation, Harris, 1926
Impact on sleep	sometimes interrupt sleep, Locke, 1677; stopped sleep, Andre, 1756
Sensory changes	Lewy Grant, 1928
Impact	Starving, Fehr and Schmidt, 1688; unable to talk, Andre, 1756; suicide, Harris, 1926

(continued)

CHAPTER 2

Table 2.1 Continued	
Trigeminal neuralgia	First descriptions, author, date
MS TN	Oppenheim, 1894; Harris, 1926; TN occurred after MS, Rushton and MacDonald, 1957
Hereditary	Lewy Grant, 1928; Patrick, 1914; Harris, 1936
Link with cardiovascular system	Lewy Grant, 1928
Link tumour	Parker, 1928
Atypical forms	Hyslop, 1936

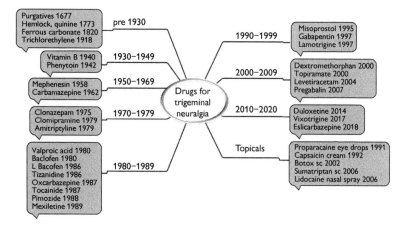

Figure 2.2 Drugs for TN
sc, subcutaneous.

2.3.2 Surgical developments

By the eighteenth century, surgical techniques were being used for alleviating the pain of TN but often resulted in severe side effects, especially sensory ones. Initial treatment was often aimed at peripheral branches but soon techniques for entering the middle fossa, and so gaining access to the Gasserian ganglion, were tried. The use of X-rays provided increased reliability of access to the ganglion just as the operating microscope made surgery in the posterior fossa so successful. In recent years, radiation techniques have been added to the neurosurgeon's armamentarium. Some of the stages in the process are shown in fig. 2.3.

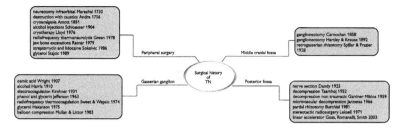

Figure 2.3 Surgery for TN

2.4 Other cranial neuralgias

Glossopharyngeal neuralgia was first described by Weisenburg in 1910 and Sicard Robineau in 1920, with Harris providing details of location and coining the current term in 1921. Hesse, in 1931, suggested that TN and glossopharyngeal neuralgia could coexist. In 1908, Ramsay Hunt discovered the correlation between herpes zoster, nervus intermedius, and geniculate neuralgia, giving his name to the syndrome.

The first description of occipital neuralgia is credited to Beruto y Lentijo and Ramos in 1821. Baillarger, in 1853, described the 'auriculotemporal syndrome' but it was not until 1923 that the neuralgia was recognized as a distinct entity by Lucie Frey, who first proposed a pathophysiological hypothesis for the pain. The first case of great auricular neuralgia was described in 1933 by Hall and that of superior laryngeal neuralgia by Tobold in 1866.

2.5 Trigeminal autonomic cephalalgias

Other episodic unilateral facial pains are classified in a group known as the trigeminal autonomic cephalalgias (TACs). The best known in this group is cluster headache which may already have been described in 1745 but the definitive description is credited to Horton in 1939 and the name to Kunkle in 1952.

The first cases of short-lasting unilateral neuralgiform headache with conjunctival injection and tearing (SUNCT) were described by Sjaastad in the late 1970s and in the 2000s it was suggested that there could be other local autonomic features, hence the name short-lasting unilateral neuralgiform headache with autonomic symptoms (SUNA). These may constitute the same condition. Paroxysmal and chronic hemicrania were found to be exquisitely responsive to indomethacin and were described in the 1970s and 1980s by Sjaastad.

2.6 Classification

In 1979, Bonica suggested that a taxonomy of pain was needed and he set up the Task Force on Taxonomy of the International Association for the Study of

Table 2.2 Development of the classification systems for headaches and orofacial pain

Year	Classification body	Title and edition
1979	IASP	Pain terms: a list with definitions and notes on usage
1986	IASP	Classification of Chronic Pain
1988	IHS	ICHD, 1st edition
1992	Dworkin/LeResche	RDC/TMD
1994	IASP	Classification of Chronic Pain, 2nd edition (updated 2011, 2012)
2003	Burchiel	Classification for facial pain: seven diagnostic labels
2004	IHS	ICHD, 2nd edition
2008	International RDC/TMD Consortium Network	RDC/TMD revised
2013	AAOP	1st Assessment, Orofacial Pain: Guidelines for Diagnosis and Management, updated four times
2013	IHS	ICHD, 3rd edition (beta version)
2018	IHS	ICHD, 3rd edition
2019	WHO	ICD-11, Chronic secondary headache or orofacial pain
2020	ICOP	International Classification of Orofacial Pain, 1st edition

AAOP, American Academy of Orofacial Pain; IASP, International Association for the Study of Pain; ICHD, International Classification of Headache Disorders; ICD-11, International Classification of Diseases, eleventh revision; ICOP, International Classification of Orofacial Pain; IHS, International Headache Society; RDC/TMD, Research Diagnostic Criteria for Temporomandibular Disorders; WHO, World Health Organization.

Pain (IASP). Interestingly, the starting point was the use of an orofacial pain taxonomy which had been set up in 1974 by the US National Institute of Dental Research. This then led to the International Headache Society putting forward its classification for head and orofacial pain. It is only recently that the International Classification of Diseases, eleventh revision (ICD-11) has included all forms of pain including orofacial pain (Table 2.2).

Most of the classifications are based on diagnostic criteria suggested by experts, but ones based on cluster analysis or ontological principles would be most useful but require considerable work. In the future, artificial intelligence which enables collection of 'big data' may help in this process.

2.7 Lay summary

TN has been known for centuries but the first descriptions that remain valid to date are those by John Fothergill in 1783. The chance naming of the condition as a form of epilepsy led to the use of a wide range of antiepileptic drugs which are still being used today. Since 1730 surgical techniques have been evolving. Initially, treatments were located at the end branches of the nerve but then moved on to the Gasserian ganglion, the point at which all three branches come together. With the advent of the operating microscope, it became possible to carry out effective surgery within the skull close to the point at which the nerve enters the brain. For patients, clinicians, and researchers to be able to communicate better about conditions, internationally agreed classification system are needed. There are now several in use and there is good agreement between them.

2.8 RECOMMENDED READING

International Classification of Orofacial Pain, 1st edition (ICOP). Cephalalgia. 2020;**40**:129–221. doi: 10.1177/0333102419893823

Klasser GD, Manfredini D, Goulet JP, et al. Oro-facial pain and temporomandibular disorders classification systems: a critical appraisal and future directions. J Oral Rehabil. 2018;**45**:258–68. doi: 10.1111/joor.12590

Penman J. Trigeminal neuralgia. In: Vinken PJ, Bruyn GN, editors. Handbook of Clinical Neurology. Amsterdam: Elsevier Science; 1968, pp. 269–322.

Stookey B, Ransohoff J. Trigeminal Neuralgia: Its History and Treatments. Springfield, IL: Charles C. Thomas; 1959.

2.9 Continuing professional development

1. Who provided the first comprehensive description of TN?
2. Why were antiepileptics chosen as a treatment?
3. Which classification system would you use for TN?

CHAPTER 3

Review of anatomy and physiology of the face in view of pain-generating and pain-mediating mechanisms

Mark Obermann

Genetics
Ze'ev Seltzer and Scott R. Diehl

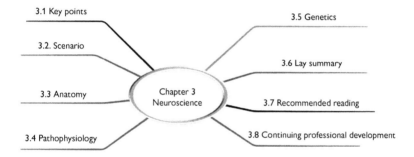

Figure 3.1 Plan of chapter

3.1 KEY POINTS

1. Peripheral innervation of the face and head is conveyed through trigeminal, glossopharyngeal, and intermedius nerves, and via occipital and great auricular nerves arising from C2–C3 roots.

2. Within the central nervous system, axon terminals from these nerves converge onto neurons in the brainstem spinal trigeminal nucleus (STN), where afferent inputs undergo the first stage of analysis by a local network of excitatory and inhibitory interneurons. Their output feeds ascending projection neurons to thalamic neurons and thence to somatosensory and associate cortices.

3. These ascending pathways are under facilitatory and inhibitory controls mediated by descending pain modulation pathways that originate in the cortex and several brainstem nuclei including periaqueductal grey, raphe

magnus, and locus coeruleus, and are additionally modulated by activity in the hypothalamus.

4. A trigeminal root lesion from neurovascular compression or other sources leads to ectopic hyperexcitability of injured primary nociceptors, to abnormal changes in the phenotype of non-nociceptive afferents to a nociceptive phenotype, and to 'central sensitization' of nociceptive projection neurons in the nucleus caudalis of the STN, manifesting in spontaneous activity and augmented response to sensory stimuli. The paroxysmal nature of pain is provisionally explained by the 'ignition hypothesis'.

5. Parasympathetic activation driven mostly by output of hyperexcited STN projection neurons causes lacrimation and rhinorrhoea in trigeminal autonomic cephalalgias.

6. Evidence suggests that most trigeminal neuralgia (TN) patients inherit very rare mutations in multiple genes important for neuronal development and maintenance, peripheral and central neuronal excitability and synaptic inhibition, myelin formation and maintenance, and other functions.

7. The rarity of TN is explained, in part, by the need for rare co-occurrent breakdowns in several nodes of the trigeminal pain network. Subtypes of TN that differ by sex, age when the condition starts, and presence of a neurovascular compression, may be explained by patients carrying mutations in different functional types of genes such as those involved with ion channels, myelination, neurotransmitters and receptors, neuronal development, etc. Some of these TN genes are aetiologically important for other craniofacial neuralgias or chronic pain elsewhere in the body.

3.2 Scenario

A pharmaceutical company is hoping that genetics will become a new approach for treatment for trigeminal neuralgia (TN). Is this worth exploring?

- Focus on abnormal afferent inputs from cranial nerves V, VII, IX, cervical nerve roots C1–C3, and autonomic pathways; disruptions in their course and innervation territories.
- Consider pathophysiological mechanisms in central pain pathways (including pain modulatory networks).
- Recall known pathophysiology of cranial neuralgias, neuropathies, and trigeminal autonomic cephalalgias (TACs) (summarized in section 3.4).
- Assess emerging knowledge of gene mutations associated with cranial neuralgias.

3.3 Anatomy

3.3.1 General

The *trigeminal nerve* is a mixed cranial nerve (CN) consisting of sensory and motor fibres. It is the main sensory nerve of the face and has three branches or divisions: (1) ophthalmic division (CN V1), (2) maxillary division (CN V2), and (3) mandibular division (CN V3) (fig. 3.2). The cutaneous innervation territories are relatively sharply demarcated with little overlap (fig. 3.3).

The cell bodies of the axons running in the three branches reside in the semilunar (Gasserian or trigeminal ganglion) in Meckel's cave where they are each enveloped by a number of satellite glial cells. CN V1 and CN V2 enter the cavernous sinus; CN V1 leaves the skull through the superior orbital fissure, and CN V2 through the foramen rotundum. CN V3 leaves the skull through the foramen ovale. The central terminals of the trigeminal neurons form the sensory root, connecting the ganglion and the brainstem, and traverse the pons to arrive at the sensory nuclei of the trigeminal brainstem nuclear complex: main sensory (pontine trigeminal), mesencephalic, and spinal trigeminal nucleus (STN). The STN extends the entire length of the medulla oblongata (fig. 3.4).

Trigeminal afferents conveying neural information evoked by noxious, innocuous, and body temperature travel down alongside the STN with the ophthalmic division fibres situated posteromedially, mandibular division fibres anterolaterally, and maxillary division fibres in the middle. Once they enter the STN and synapse with interneurons in the trigeminal nucleus (pars) caudalis in the caudal part of the STN, a new somatotopic arrangement is formed that resembles that of onion skin with the perioral area represented rostrally and the lateral face caudally. The trigeminal nucleus caudalis also receives inputs from the glossopharyngeal, intermedius, and vagal nerves as well as C2–C3 spinal nerves. These afferent inputs, together with local interneurons, projection neurons of ascending pain pathways, and terminal arborizations of neurons descending from the cortex, thalamus, hypothalamus, and brainstem nuclei of the descending pain modulation system, constitute a neural assembly referred to as the trigeminocervical complex (TCC). This convergence of afferents from multiple sources explains the phenomenon of referred pain from the head and neck, and trigeminal autonomic reflex (fig. 3.5 and fig. 3.6).

The trigeminal motor nucleus in the pons tegmentum receives sensory input from central projections of the trigeminal (and other cranial) nerves via segmental interneurons. Axons from the motor nucleus travel through the pons and exit as the motor root on the medial aspect of the trigeminal sensory root. They pass deep to the trigeminal ganglion in Meckel's cave and for a short distance join the sensory axons in the mandibular nerve (fig. 3.2).

The trigeminal nerve does not have parasympathetic fibres but is closely associated with parasympathetic ganglia along its course. CN V1 is associated with the ciliary ganglion where fibres supply the ciliary and sphincter pupillae

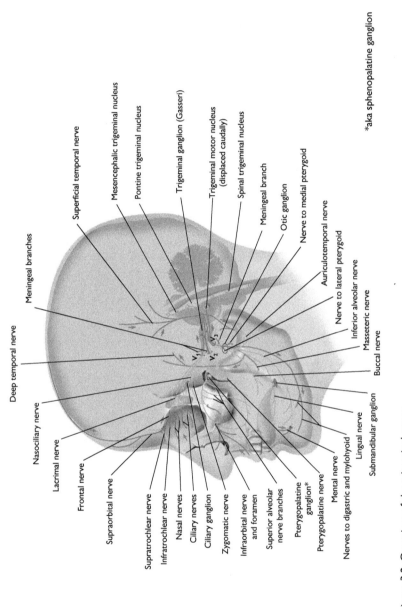

Figure 3.2 Overview of the trigeminal nerve

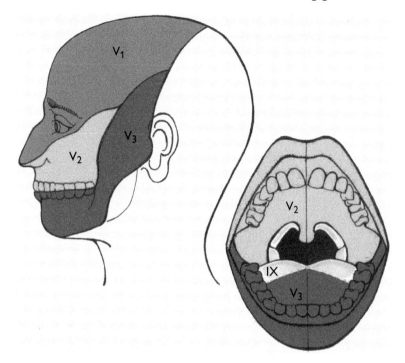

Figure 3.3 Sensory innervation territories of the ophthalmic (V₁), maxillary (V₂), and mandibular (V₃) branches of the trigeminal nerve as well as the glossopharyngeal nerve (IX, intraoral)

Reproduced from Cruccu G, Finnerup NB, Jensen TS, et al. Neurology 2016;87:220-8. doi: 10.1212/WNL.0000000000002840 with permission from Wolters Kluwer Health, Inc.

muscles via the short ciliary nerve. CN V3 is associated with fibres from the otic ganglion innervating the parotid gland as well as from the submandibular ganglion whose fibres form the chorda tympani running along CN V3, before entering the lingual nerve. CN V2 is associated with the sphenopalatine (pterygopalatine) ganglion which innervates the lacrimal, the palatal, and the nasal mucous glands (fig. 3.2).

The *glossopharyngeal nerve* (CN IX) is a mixed nerve that contains sensory, motor, and parasympathetic fibres. It leaves the rostral medulla of the pons as rootlets which soon converge into a nerve that leaves the cranium through the jugular foramen (fig. 3.7).

Primary glossopharyngeal afferents convey nociceptive and thermoceptive inputs from the posterior third of the tongue, oropharynx, middle ear, and mastoid cells (fig. 3.3 and fig. 3.7). Afferents innervating the posterior third of the tongue

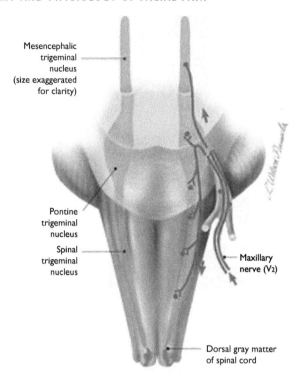

Mesencephalic trigeminal nucleus (size exaggerated for clarity)

Pontine trigeminal nucleus

Spinal trigeminal nucleus

Maxillary nerve (V₂)

Dorsal gray matter of spinal cord

Figure 3.4 Trigeminal brainstem nuclear complex

Ventral view of the brainstem. Note the extension of the spinal trigeminal nucleus (STN) caudally.

Reproduced from Wilson-Pauwels L., Stewart P., Akersson E., Spacey S., eds., Cranial Nerves 3rd Edition. (2010 PMPH-USA) with permission from PMPH-USA.

carry information on tastants, and from the carotid body. The cell bodies of these neurons are located in the superior or inferior glossopharyngeal ganglion, which lie just outside the jugular foramen and their central processes terminate in the caudal STN. Cell bodies of afferents from taste receptors and the carotid sinus and body are located in the inferior ganglion and their central processes reach the solitary nucleus in the rostral medulla oblongata. Axons from the medullary nucleus ambiguus give rise to motor fibres travelling in the glossopharyngeal nerve, to innervate the stylopharyngeal and superior pharyngeal constrictor muscles. Parasympathetic preganglionic fibres originating from the salivatory nucleus in the medulla travel in CN IX to the otic ganglion, from which the postganglionic fibres supply the parotid gland (fig. 3.7).

The *intermedius nerve* is considered part of the facial nerve, because it travels closely attached to the latter and joins it in the internal acoustic meatus. It consists

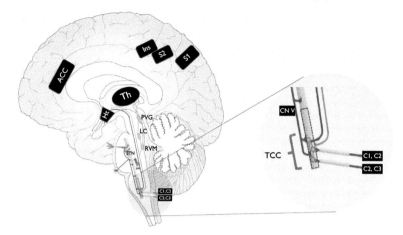

Figure 3.5 Trigeminal central pain pathways

The central terminals of the first-order trigeminal nociceptors synapse on interneurons in the caudal part of STN where also C1, C2, and C3 afferents terminate. From this assembly (TCC, trigeminocervical complex) bidirectional connections exist with a number of midbrain centres, notably hypothalamus (Ht), thalamus (TH), and periaqueductal grey (PAG). The main set of ascending fibres (indicated in red) travel in the ventral and dorsal trigeminothalamic tracts to reach the ventroposteromedial thalamus (VPM) nucleus where they synapse on interneurons. From the VPM nucleus third-order neurones project to somatosensory cortices (S1, S2), insula, and limbic areas involved in processing of nociceptive input. Conscious pain experience is associated with an interaction of several brain networks working in parallel (not shown). The ACC is a key structure contributing to the activation of the descending pain modulation which involves thalamus, PAG, nucleus locus coeruleus (LC), and rostroventromedial medulla (RVM) from where the tracts (shown in green) descend to supply the TCC. Descending modulation involves both facilitatory and inhibitory mechanisms. Ht has efferent connections with the TCC and may explain some of the rhythmicity of trigeminal autonomic pains. (Location of nuclei and centres approximate only. Not all connections shown. See text for details.)

of three types of fibres: (1) sensory fibres carrying neural messages on tastants applied to the anterior part of the tongue and projecting to the solitary nucleus, (2) preganglionic parasympathetic fibres projecting to the sphenopalatine (pterygopalatine) and submandibular ganglia, and (3) cutaneous sensory fibres originating from the external auditory canal and projecting to the rostral part of the trigeminal spinal nucleus. Their cell bodies are in the geniculate ganglion. Sensory innervation areas include the concha, back of the ear lobe, and posterior wall of the external auditory meatus. From the geniculate ganglion, parasympathetic connections supply the lacrimal gland.

Three sensory nerves supply the occiput up to the top of the head. The *greater occipital nerve* (GON) arises from the medial branch of C2, the *lesser occipital nerve* (LON) from the dorsal branch of C2, and the *third occipital nerve* (TON) from C3 (see Chapter 13, fig. 13.1). The innervation territories of the three nerves overlap significantly and there are frequent nerve anastomoses, especially between TON (that innervates most of the posterior

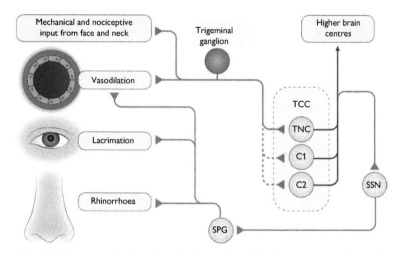

Figure 3.6 Trigeminal autonomic reflex

See text for narrative.

Reproduced from May, A., Schwedt, T., Magis, D. et al. Cluster headache. Nat Rev Dis Primers 4, 18006 (2018). https://doi.org/10.1038/nrdp.2018.6 with permission from Springer Nature

scalp), and LON (that mediates sensation from the scalp posterior to the auricle and parts of the auricle itself). TON also innervates a small cutaneous area below the nuchal line.

The *great auricular nerve*, part of the superficial cervical plexus, originates from the dorsal ramus of C2 and C3 spinal roots, and winds around the sternocleido-mastoid muscle to supply the skin over the preauricular area, parotid, jaw angle, inferior pinna, mastoid, and upper lateral neck (see Chapter 13, fig. 13.2). The *auriculotemporal nerve* is a sensory branch of the mandibular nerve and innervates the ear lobe, internal meatus, temple, preauricular skin, and temporomandibular joint capsule.

3.3.2 Central ascending trigeminal pathways

Nociceptive and thermoceptive inputs from the STN to the ventroposteromedial (VPM) nucleus of the thalamus are carried via ventral and dorsal trigeminothalamic tracts that comprise axons of second-order projection neurons whose cell bodies reside in the STN. Third-order neurons from VPM nucleus project to the ipsi-lateral postcentral gyrus where facial representation is disproportionately larger than other body parts. It is situated laterally in the primary somatosensory cortex. Some projections reach the secondary somatosensory cortex, insular cortex, and the anterior cingulate cortex (ACC).

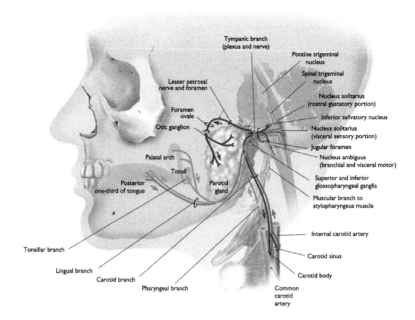

Figure 3.7 Overview of the glossopharyngeal nerve

Reproduced from Wilson-Pauwels L., Stewart P., Akersson E., Spacey S., eds., Cranial Nerves 3rd Edition. (2010 PMPH-USA) with permission from PMPH-USA.

Decoding incoming nociceptive inputs is a complex process involving several brain regions and networks. Primary and secondary somatosensory cortices, thalamus, and posterior part of the insula are involved in sensory-discriminative aspects of pain while affective-motivational components are processed in the medial pain network including the ACC, anterior insula, and amygdala. Several other brain areas are involved in motor, cognitive, and autonomic responses to noxious stimuli. The current view is that the perception of pain requires the spatiotemporal integration of parallel distributed and serial processing of noci-ceptive inputs in dedicated networks associating physical attributes of location, intensity, duration, and type with the emotive attributes of affect and suffering.

Alongside with pain processing, the ACC and central nucleus of the amyg-dala connect via the periaqueductal grey in the midbrain with brainstem nuclei involved in descending modulation, including the locus coeruleus and rostral ventromedial medulla, which send projections to the STN. Remaining under opioidergic, GABAergic and monoaminergic control, these connections are ei-ther facilitatory or inhibitory.

3.4 Pathophysiology

The complex mechanisms of neuropathic pain are only partially understood but can be summarized as hyperexcitability of certain parts of the somatosensory system due to local changes in ion channel expression, altered second-order and third-order neuron connectivity and sensitization, and dysfunctional segmental and descending modulations. These neuroplastic changes are modulated by abnormal neuroimmune regulation, altered neural–glial interactions, and involvement of the autonomic nervous system at multiple levels of the ascending sensory pathway. In cranial nerves, similarly to spinal nerves, neuronal hyperexcitability is linked to overexpression of voltage-gated calcium and sodium channels in nociceptor cell bodies and free nerve endings while expression of potassium channels is decreased. These changes manifest in ongoing spontaneous ectopic discharges in injured afferents and their cell bodies in associated ganglia, and flooding of central nervous system pain pathways with nociceptive input that is perceived as pain. At the first synapse in the central nervous system, this massive nociceptive input generates the release of glutamate and other excitatory neurotransmitters and peptidergic modulators into the synaptic cleft that increases excitability of local interneurons and second-order projection nociceptive neurons. These lead to imbalances between facilitatory and inhibitory descending modulation of segmental interneurons and projection neurons in the STN. These, and other synaptic events, cause 'central sensitization' of the STN and associated nuclei in the thalamus. The neurophysiological correlate of 'central sensitization' is a leftward shift of the stimulus–response curve that clinically corresponds to mechanical and thermal allodynia (pain in response to a normally innocuous stimulus) and hyperalgesia (increased pain in response to a normally noxious stimulus).

The above-described mechanisms offer a plausible explanation for continuous pain and sensory changes characteristic of painful neuropathies, but not for the key feature of TN, that is, sudden-onset, intense pain paroxysms, evoked by innocuous stimuli applied on small trigger zones. In classical TN, the favoured hypothesis combines the local effect of neurovascular compression and secondary hyperexcitability changes of injured axons and their cell bodies. Neurovascular compression induces local demyelination in large diameter myelinated fibres that normally convey input on innocuous stimuli such as touch, making possible a cross-excitation with closely apposed nociceptive fibres. This 'ephaptic transmission' allows touch-evoked impulses to jump from large diameter fibres to nociceptive afferents (see Seltzer and Devor, in 'Recommended reading' at the end of the chapter). Simultaneously, the epigenetically increased expression of sodium and other ion channel subunits, and their assembly in the cell bodies' outer membrane, makes them another source of ectopic spontaneous sensory input. In addition, neurons and satellite glial cells in the ganglion express gap junction proteins that when assembled in their membranes facilitate a chemical communication between the neurons and several satellite glial cells surrounding them. This leads to a cluster pool of highly excitable ganglion cells, some of which are nociceptive, easily triggered in the periphery by touch-evoked impulses. This clinically manifests as a painful paroxysm. This 'ignition hypothesis' was offered by Devor and Rappaport in 2002 but it cannot alone explain all pain paroxysms in TN. For example, when no frank neurovascular compression can be demonstrated, other mechanisms must be sought although they remain unclear (see Chapter 10). Another pathological factor, for example, genetics (see section 3.5) should be considered in the causation of TN.

The pathophysiology of TACs shares some of the features with trigeminal nerve-mediated pain. The STN (and its functional equivalent, the trigeminocervical complex) is at the centre of pain generation in all TACs. Evidence from surgical interventions suggests that pathology of the peripheral nerve is more causative in short-lasting unilateral neuralgiform headache with conjunctival injection and tearing (SUNCT)/short-lasting unilateral neuralgiform headache with autonomic symptoms (SUNA) than in other TACs (see Chapter 14). Uniquely, the activity of the STN is strongly modulated by the posterior hypothalamus in cluster headache and probably in other TACs, and could explain the temporal nature of pain attacks. The STN activates neurons in the superior salivary nucleus, which sends preganglionic fibres to the sphenopalatine ganglion, from which postganglionic projections are sent to the lacrimal glands, nasal mucosa, and multiple arteries. Activation of the trigeminal system is associated with autonomic symptoms of TACs, lacrimation, rhinorrhoea, and conjunctival injection (fig. 3.6).

3.5 Genetics

Familial aggregation, the observation that close relatives are affected by a rare disorder more often than expected by chance, is one line of evidence suggesting that a disease or disorder has a genetic (inherited) basis. We see this phenomenon occasionally for TN patients, but only rarely, and never with affected family members showing frequent transmission across multiple generations as in conditions caused by a single gene such as certain forms of colon or breast cancer, Huntington disease, and some forms of spinocerebellar ataxia. This might suggest that TN has a recessive mode of transmission such as occurs for cystic fibrosis, where only very rarely do we find multiple generations of family members affected, because it is unlikely that a spouse marrying into such a family would also carry a mutated copy of the disease gene. However, a single-gene aetiology for TN is also unlikely, because among those rare families that have a pair or more of close relatives affected by TN, they often exhibit transmission across generations, consistent with dominant transmission. A third possibility for the genetic basis of TN risk is that the condition usually only develops when damaging mutations occur at a few or up to a dozen genes that play important roles in several biological pathways (called 'oligogenic' inheritance, literally 'a few genes'). If this mechanism is at work for most cases of TN, this would explain why the condition is so rare, since TN would occur only when a person carries a specific combination of mutated genes. It would also explain why we only very rarely observe

TN transmitted across multiple generations, because family members in the later generations would most likely not inherit all of the necessary mutations that their TN-affected relative inherited.

Since we believe that gene mutations are important risk factors for developing TN, the next important question is 'What kinds of genes are they?' As TN is known to be associated with neurovascular compression of the trigeminal nerve, it is possible that some people have inherited genes that make it more likely that blood vessels develop over time in a tortuous way that leads to nerve compression. Alternatively, however, this may be simply an inevitable result of ageing and not strongly influenced by a person's genetic makeup. This leads us to consider a very large number of genes that affect development and cellular functioning of neurons and glia. Possibilities range from peripheral receptors of primary afferents, to myelin formation surrounding some axons and their maintenance and repair following injury, as well as genes encoding ion channels and other electrogenic mechanisms that underlie neuronal excitability. Excitatory and inhibitory synaptic neurotransmitters and their receptors in the STN and higher up along the trigeminal pain network may also be involved. There are hundreds of different ion channel genes alone, and scientists are still at an early stage of understanding how they interact in normal conditions as well as how they may cause loss of normal function when combinations of mutations are present. If, as we have suggested here, TN is caused by various mutations in multiple genes involving different functional nodes of the trigeminal pain network, it will be necessary to obtain the DNA sequence of all such genes in many TN patients (as well as other forms of neuropathic pain) to fully elucidate the complex processes involved. Only in very recent years has gene sequencing technology advanced to a state where it is cost-feasible to undertake such large-scale studies and early results now emerging appear to be consistent with the multiple rare mutation model of TN aetiology, as we suggest here.

Finally, aside from the presence or absence of neurovascular compression, it is often assumed that all TN patients share the same causal mechanisms. Based on what we see for other neurological disorders such as the epilepsies, Charcot–Marie–Tooth disease, or other ataxias, this assumption seems unlikely to hold for TN and other forms of craniofacial pain. It is far more likely that subgroups of TN patients exist that have different causal genetic mechanisms. For example, female patients with TN pain onset at a relatively young age of less than 45 years old without neurovascular compression may have a very different suite of gene mutations than older patients with severe neurovascular compression of both sexes. If this turns out to be the case, then it logically follows that the most effective pharmacological (or other means of treatment) may not be the same for the different aetiological subgroups. In order for a clinician to provide each of their patients with the best therapy available, it may be necessary to base the treatment decisions on knowledge of each patient's set of causative mutations rather than using the 'trial and error' and 'one size fits all' methods of treatment available today.

CHAPTER 3

3.6 Lay summary

Please look at the figures to improve your understanding of the text. Three cranial nerves and upper cervical nerve roots convey nociceptive input (signals sent by specific pain receptors, or nociceptors) from the face and head. Their fibres converge on a dedicated ensemble of nerve cells and glial cells (protective and supportive cells) in the lower part of the brainstem, called the STN. From there, nociceptive input is transmitted to the brain where it is processed to create the conscious awareness of pain and determine its location, quality, and intensity as well the emotional response. To this end, the brain communicates with the STN, modifying its activity on demand. The STN indirectly controls the autonomic nervous system responsible for many symptoms in TACs. In some cases, TN is caused by root compression; in other cases, the cause is unknown. But a compression of the root is also seen in many healthy people who are asymptomatic. This leads us to propose a genetic model for the causation of TN that combines gene mutations of two types: one that controls the risk for root compression and a separate one that controls TN symptoms. Moreover, it now appears likely that TN (and some of the other forms of chronic craniofacial pain disorders) are caused in a large part by rare, so-called damaging mutations in multiple genes that are normally expressed in neural and glial cells of the trigeminal pain network. Each patient may have inherited several damaged genes, and different subgroups of patients may have inherited different kinds of genes with diverse biological functions. In the future, a complete understanding of how inherited genetic variation causes TN may enable clinicians to provide their patients with optimal therapies targeted to address each individual patient's profile of mutations.

3.7 RECOMMENDED READING

Dong W, Jin SC, Allocco A, et al. Exome sequencing implicates impaired GABA signaling and neuronal ion transport in trigeminal neuralgia. iScience. 2020;23:101552. doi: 10.1016/j.isci.2020.101552

Gambeta E, Chichorro JG, Zamponi GW. Trigeminal neuralgia: an overview from pathophysiology to pharmacological treatments. Mol Pain. 2020;16:1–18 doi: 10.1177/1744806920901890

Giani L, Proietti Cecchini A, Leone M. Cluster headache and TACS: state of the art. Neurol Sci. 2020;41 Suppl 2:367–75. doi: 10.1007/s10072-020-04639-4

Seltzer Z, Devor M. Ephaptic transmission in chronically damaged peripheral nerves. Neurology. 1979;29:1061–4. doi: 10.1212/wnl.29.7.1061

Smith CA, Paskhover B, Mammis A. Molecular mechanisms of trigeminal neuralgia: a systematic review. Clin Neurol Neurosurg. 2021;200:106397. doi: 10.1016/j.clineuro.2020.106397

For online learning go to, for example: https://www.kenhub.com/en/library/anatomy/the-trigeminal-nerve

3.8 Continuing professional development

1. For unilateral pain in and around the ear, which nerve(s) could be involved?
2. Explain the functional significance of the caudal part of the STN in nociception.
3. How are genetic factors implicated in familial and non-familial TN?

CHAPTER 4

Epidemiology of trigeminal neuralgia and its variants

Vishal R. Aggarwal and Joanna M. Zakrzewska

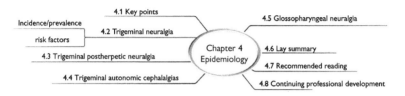

Figure 4.1 Plan of chapter

4.1 KEY POINTS

1. Trigeminal neuralgia and its variants are rare with prevalence in the range of 0.1–0.7%.
2. Variations outside this prevalence range are due to inconsistencies in disease definition and case ascertainment.
3. Future epidemiological studies need to ensure consistency in disease definition.
4. Aetiological factors and disease burden need further investigation through high-quality, prospective, population-based studies.

4.2 Trigeminal neuralgia

4.2.1 Global prevalence and sex distribution

Trigeminal neuralgia (TN) is considered to be a rare disease with a prevalence in the range of 0.1–0.7% (Table 4.1). There has been one systematic review of the prevalence of TN in the population and it included three studies that were population based and are presented in Table 4.1. A further systematic review by Van Hecke and colleagues on the epidemiology of neuropathic pain in the general population included seven studies dealing with TN.

Other studies have used convenience rather than population samples and these have reported similar or lower prevalence to population studies. On the whole, prevalence of TN is similar across global regions as shown in Table 4.1.

Table 4.1 Epidemiology of trigeminal neuralgia

Country	Sample type size	Years	No. of cases	Prevalence	95% CI	Incidence	95% CI	Comments	Reference
USA, Rochester		1945–1956				4/100,000			Kurland 1958; doi: 10.1016/ 0021-9681(58)90002-x
USA, Rochester	Mayo Clinic medical records, population of 752,629	1945–1969	36			4.0/100,000	2.7–5.3	More women, estimate 5000–10,000 new cases a year in USA, linked to multiple sclerosis	Yoshimasu et al. 1972; doi: 10.1212/ wnl.22.9.952
USA, Massachusetts General Hospital	Hospital, surgically managed 526, controls with spine disorders 528	1955–1970	140			2.96/100,000 males 3.47/100,000 females		More women, numbers start to rise from 55 years	Rothman & Monson 1973; doi: 10.1016/ 0021-9681(73)90075-1
USA,* Rochester	Hospital data	1945–1984	75			4.7/100,000			Katusic et al. 1990; doi: 10.1002/ana.410270114
UK, Carlisle	GP & hospital records, Carlisle population 71,101	1955–1961	10			2.1/100,000			Brewis et al. 1966; PMID: 4224973
UK, London*	GP & hospital, London 100,230	Jan 1995– July 1996				8/100,000		Age/sex adjusted	Macdonald et al. 2000; doi: 10.1093/brain/ 123.4.665

Country	Source	Period	Number	Rate	Incidence	Range	Notes	Reference
UK*	GP records, General Practice Research Database 6.8 million	Jan 1992–April 2002	8268	24.8/10,000	26.8/100,000	26.2–27.4	Included drugs used not validated	Hall et al. 2006; doi: 10.1016/j.pain.2006.01.030
UK*	GP records, General Practice Research Database 2.9 million	May 2002–July 2005	1862		27.3/100,000			Hall et al. 2008; doi: 10.1186/1471-2296-9-26
France	Questionnaire, town 993	1984	1	0.1			Neurological disease main focus	Munoz et al. 1988; PMID: 3262231
Norway**	Face-to-face interview, Vågå city 1838 of population 2074	2000	2	0.16	0.03–0.40 calculated by De Toledo		Age 18–65, both women, ophthalmic and mandibular	Sjaastad & Bakketeig 2007; doi: 10.1007/s10194-006-0292-4
Holland*	GP records 362,693	Jan 1996–Dec 2003	322		28.9/100,000 person years	25.8–32.1	Neuropathic pain	Dieleman et al. 2008; doi: 10.1016/j.pain.2008.03.002
Holland*	GP records 479,949	Jan 1996–Sept 2006	118		12.6/100,000	10.5–15.1	Before validation 21.7 higher women, only facial pain	Koopman et al. 2009; doi: 10.1016/j.pain.2009.08.023
Holland*	GP records 5273 varicella and 3371 had herpes zoster	2004–2008	75		0.009%/population/year***		TN reported as a complication of HZ	Pierek et al. 2012; doi: 10.1186/1471-2334-12-110

(continued)

Table 4.1 Continued

Country	Sample type size	Years	No. of cases	Prevalence	95% CI	Incidence	95% CI	Comments	Reference
Germany**	Questionnaire, population town 6000	2001–2002	10	0.3	0.1–0.5			Interviewed positives, some controls, part of a headache survey but this was on facial pain age 18 to >65 TN cases 42–67 years, 7 women 3 men	Mueller et al. 2011; doi: 10.1177/0333102411424619
Italy	Bruneck study Population of one village 13,534 Selected 40–79-year-olds, 4793 in 1990 Follow-up in 2005 for 55–94-year-olds	2005	9	1.6% lifetime Men 0.8%, women 2.3%	0.6–2.6			Interviewed more women >75 years (6 of the cases), lowest in 55–64 years, 1 case of symptomatic TN	Schwaiger et al. 2008; doi: 10.1111/j.1468-2982.2008.01705.x
Egypt**	Door-to-door interviews using standardized Arabic questionnaire, population city 33,285, sample size 13,541	June 2010–Jan 2012	4	29.5/100,000 age specific Calculated by De Toledo 0.03 (0.01–0.08)	22.3–34.7			All females >37, 3 depression neurologists did MRIs	El-Tallawy et al. 2013; doi: 10.1016/j.clineuro.2013.04.014

CI, confidence interval.

* Included in van Hecke et al. systematic review; ** included in De Toledo systematic review; *** calculated as 75/165,000 over 5-year period.

Penman estimated the annual prevalence based on indirect calculations on the number of patients with multiple sclerosis and estimated 4.7 per 1 million men and 7.2 per 1 million women. Most studies report a higher incidence in women, with a female-to-male ratio varying from 1.5:1 to 1.8:1. In the German cohort study (population of 6000) based on initial questionnaires and then face-to-face interviews of the ten identified TN patients, only one had been correctly diagnosed prior to the study. Seven of the ten cases were female. The study authors think this could have been an underestimate as patients with head and face pain may have been more willing to complete the questionnaire. They put the true estimate at 0.16–0.3%.

The Bruneck study in Italy was a population-based study that found nine cases of TN; one was symptomatic and six of the cases were in women aged over 75 years. This made a lifetime prevalence of 1.6%; for women it was 2% and for men 1.2%. This is higher than in any other series and could be due to the older age of the study population. The prevalence of all primary headaches was 51.7% but no trigeminal autonomic cephalalgias were found. This study also included health-related quality of life which was worse in the TN patients (mean 53.6 for cases compared to 17.3 for controls) and after adjustment for age, sex, and social status was significant (p <0.001).

TN is very rare in children and adolescents and patients under 25 years of age have been noted to have poorer outcomes after microvascular decompression than older people.

4.2.2 Aetiology and risk factors

The disease most frequently linked with TN is multiple sclerosis (in around 5–10% of cases). A very small percentage may have tumours, mostly benign. Hypertension is a risk factor and strokes are more likely. Data from a population-based study in Taiwan highlights an increased risk of depression, anxiety, and sleep disorders after a diagnosis of TN. This was also found in a population-based study in Egypt where three of the four identified cases had depression.

4.3 Trigeminal postherpetic neuralgia and herpes zoster

This is a rare condition that develops more than 6 months after an acute herpes zoster (HZ) infection. Of all cases of HZ, 12–25% involve the trigeminal or facial nerves. The ophthalmic (V1) branch is affected in 60–92% (HZ ophthalmicus). The incidence of HZ ophthalmicus prior to the introduction of vaccination was reported to be 31 per 100,000 person-years. Pain lasts longer than 3 months in 3–52% of patients after acute HZ (postherpetic neuralgia); once established, it will last for more than a year in 20–50%. These figures are likely to be significantly influenced in the future by expanding population-based vaccination programmes. Vaccination has been shown to reduce the incidence of HZ by 35% and postherpetic neuralgia by 50%.

4.4 Trigeminal autonomic cephalalgias

Cluster headache has a prevalence of about 0.1%. The peak age of onset is between the third and fourth decades and is four times more common in men. It is often associated with smokers and there is a strong family history.

There is little prevalence data on paroxysmal hemicrania in the population and it is estimated to be 0.05% in the age range of 18–65 years. There appears to be a slight predominance of women and this occurs in older people in the fourth and fifth decades. No population-based studies or estimates are available for hemicrania continua, but it is believed to be equally rare with a similar demographic distribution as paroxysmal hemicrania. In one study from a dedicated headache pain clinic, 0.4% of new patients seen were diagnosed as having hemicrania continua. Future epidemiological studies of paroxysmal hemicrania and hemicrania continua will have to overcome the challenge of confirmation of the diagnosis by a positive indomethacin test (see Chapter 14).

Short-lasting unilateral neuralgiform headache attacks with conjunctival injection and tearing (SUNCT) and short-lasting unilateral neuralgiform headache attacks with cranial autonomic features (SUNA) may not be as rare as initially estimated, 6.6/100,000, but as high as 109/100,000 and 240/100,000, respectively. Recent large series show a female predominance and although reported in infancy, its peak is in the fifth decade.

4.5 Glossopharyngeal neuralgia

Estimates have suggested an incidence of 0.8 per 100,000 population and, like TN, a slight increase in women.

4.6 Lay summary

TN, a condition characterized by intense electric shock-like pain in the face, is rare with 0.1–0.7% of the population reporting it at any point in time. Thus, for a population of 60 million we would expect there to be about 60,000 cases of TN. The cause of this condition is not well understood and currently we know that people with multiple sclerosis have a higher risk of developing TN. Cases of TN are also more common in those with high blood pressure. This condition imposes an immense burden on patients who have an increased risk of depression, anxiety, and sleep disorders after diagnosis. Future high-quality studies are needed to understand the causes and burden of TN so that we can improve outcomes for those suffering from this debilitating condition.

4.7 RECOMMENDED READING

De Toledo IP, Conti Réus J, Fernandes M, et al. Prevalence of trigeminal neuralgia: a systematic review. J Am Dent Assoc. 2016;147:570–6. doi: 10.1016/j.adaj.2016.02.014

Fischera M, Marziniak M, Gralow I, et al. The incidence and prevalence of cluster headache: a meta-analysis of population-based studies. Cephalalgia. 2008;28:614–8. doi: 10.1111/j.1468-2982.2008.01592.x

Katusic S, Williams DB, Beard CM, et al Epidemiology and clinical features of idiopathic trigeminal neuralgia and glossopharyngeal neuralgia: similarities and differences, Rochester, Minnesota, 1945–1984. Neuroepidemiology. 1991;10:276–81. doi: 10.1159/000110284.

Kawai K, Gebremeskel BG, Acosta CJ. Systematic review of incidence and complications of herpes zoster: towards a global perspective. BMJ Open. 2014;4:e004833. doi:10.1136/bmjopen-2014-004833

Lambru G, Rantell K, Levy A, et al. A prospective comparative study and analysis of predictors of SUNA and SUNCT. Neurology. 2019;93:e1127–37. doi:10.1212/WNL.0000000000008134

Pan SL, Chen LS, Yen MF, et al. Increased risk of stroke after trigeminal neuralgia—a population-based follow-up study. Cephalalgia. 2011;31:937–42. doi: 10.1177/0333102411405225

Pan SL, Yen MF, Chiu YH, et al. Increased risk of trigeminal neuralgia after hypertension: a population-based study. Neurology. 2011;77:1605–10. doi: 10.1212/WNL.0b013e3182343354

van Hecke O, Austin SK, Khan RA, et al. Neuropathic pain in the general population: a systematic review of epidemiological studies. Pain. 2014;155:654–62. doi: 10.1016/j.pain.2013.11.013

Wu TH, Hu LY, Lu T, et al. Risk of psychiatric disorders following trigeminal neuralgia: a nationwide population-based retrospective cohort study. J Headache Pain. 2015;16:64. doi: 10.1186/s10194-015-0548-y

4.8 Continuing professional development

1. Why are there variations in the prevalence of TN?
2. What are the risk factors for TN?
3. Which of the trigeminal autonomic cephalalgias is most prevalent?

General approach to diagnosis and assessment of the facial pain patient

Diagnosis
Joanna M. Zakrzewska and Turo Nurmikko

Imaging
Mojgan Hodaie and Karen D. Davis

Neurophysiological testing
Gianfranco De Stefano and Andrea Truini

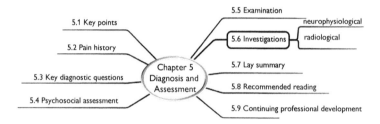

Figure 5.1 Plan of chapter

5.1 KEY POINTS

1. Clinicians seeing patients with facial pain should obtain a comprehensive clinical, family, and social history which can take time.
2. A possible diagnosis of a cranial neuralgia can be deduced from eight key questions.
3. Validated questionnaires to measure pain, affect, interference, and quality of life are useful in establishing the pain's impact at baseline and subsequent visits.
4. Clinical examination may provide a few further helpful details.
5. Magnetic resonance imaging is the most advanced method for establishing the aetiology of clinically established trigeminal and other cranial neuralgias and neuropathies.
6. Specific three-dimensional reconstruction sequences are used to visualize the root entry zone, trigeminal nerve, and surrounding vasculature. Other sequences are used to show multiple sclerosis or single pontine lesions.

7. Diffusion tensor imaging is a promising tool for investigation of microstructural changes in the affected nerve(s).
8. Trigeminal reflex testing is abnormal in secondary trigeminal neuralgia and trigeminal neuropathy; useful for patients who cannot undergo magnetic resonance imaging.

5.2 Pain history

Assessment of a patient with craniofacial pain may seem a trivial task but in actuality poses a formidable challenge. There is a bewildering range of painful conditions affecting the head and, given that currently there are no reliable biomarkers for pain, the history elicited from the patient remains decisive. And while the pain description is an instrumental part of the history, its significance cannot be fully understood without taking into account relevant medical, psychological, cultural, ethnic, and social factors that influence the patient's pain experience. A patient-centred assessment that follows a biopsychosocial framework (where all three components are explored) has the best chance of grasping the patient's problem accurately. In this context it is crucial that patients are given time to tell their story and that clinicians give their full attention to the narrative that unfolds. (This issue is discussed in detail in Chapter 16.)

There are published guidelines that both define the standards for acceptable practice and offer guidance on how to achieve them within the patient–clinician consultation. As an example, a Faculty of Pain Medicine (UK) document entitled 'Conducting Quality Consultation in Pain Medicine (2018)' provides useful background reading and a reminder of the complex skills required for successful consultations (https://fpm.ac.uk/sites/fpm/files/documents/2019-08/Conducting%20Quality%20Consultations%202018.pdf). The appendix contains details on different models that can be used to facilitate healthcare consultations on all kinds of pain.

5.3 Eight-question approach to the diagnosis of cranial neuralgia

While recognizing the importance of the impact of pain on the patient's emotional well-being, functionality, and quality of life, it is critical that the clinician gets a full understanding of its physical details. An interview technique that is based on open-ended questions will go a long way but occasional prompting will be appropriate as long as care is taken not to lead the narrative. At the end of the interview, one should have a good understanding of the characteristics of the pain: its quality, intensity, location, temporal aspects, aggravating and attenuating factors, associated symptoms, and impact on the patient's life (fig. 5.2). As will be emphasized repeatedly throughout this book, it is the detailed history that allows a meaningful diagnosis to be made.

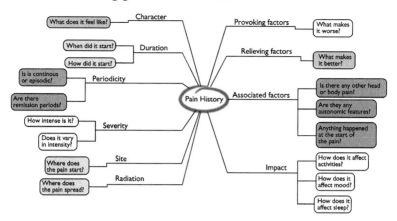

Figure 5.2 Key features of a pain history
Some key questions that should be asked.

Clinical examination in many cases serves more to confirm than detect, although it has a role in distinguishing two similar conditions. Imaging or neurophysiological and laboratory tests are used to establish (or rule out) a specific aetiology and are useful only if the clinically established diagnosis is accurate. Each cranial neuralgia tends to respond selectively to a limited number of treatment regimens and this necessitates a secure diagnosis for the best treatment outcome. In contrast, proceeding with an appropriate intervention for one condition (e.g. percutaneous trigeminal rhizolysis for trigeminal neuralgia (TN)) may significantly worsen a similar pain with slightly different presentation (trigeminal neuropathy). To help them to remember what details of pain students should query they often are taught a mnemonic: SOCRATES (Site, onset, character, radiation, alleviating factors, timing, exacerbating factors, severity)

Here we present a modification of it, a set of questions and an algorithm-based decision tree—not a mnemonic, rather a list of easily memorable binary questions that the clinician can ask during the interview (fig. 5.3). Suitable for chronic or long-standing craniofacial pain, it is constructed to illustrate how a methodical stepwise application of pain-related key questions and answers helps the clinician to reach a precision diagnosis of a cranial neuralgia. It is presented here to help the readers familiarize themselves with the questioning strategy—a tool for training and not for rigid implementation in the clinic.

5.3.1 Diagnostic decision tree for cranial neuralgias

See fig. 5.3.

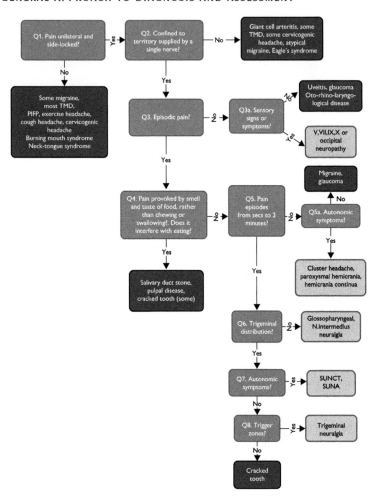

Figure 5.3 Diagnostic decision tree

Question 1. Is the pain unilateral and side-locked?

Cranial neuralgias, neuropathies, and trigeminal autonomic cephalalgias (TACs) are nearly always unilateral and side-locked, while most headaches and painful ophthalmic and otorhinolaryngological pain conditions are not. Bilateral craniofacial pain is almost always nociceptive or nociplastic, not neuropathic. Atypical migraine, giant cell arteritis, neck and pharyngeal malignancies, and glaucoma may present as unilateral pain, but these conditions will be ruled out as the interview continues. In contrast, it is exceptional for a cranial neuralgia to present as bilateral facial pain. With TN it happens rarely, and usually in people with multiple sclerosis, but with one side clearly affected first.

Decision tree

If the answer is Yes, proceed to Question 2. If the answer is No, consider diagnostic alternatives suggested in the decision tree. If the answer is unequivocal, go to Question 2.

Question 2. Is the pain confined to a territory innervated by a single nerve?

The origin of practically all cranial neuralgias and TACs can be tracked down to the dysfunction of a single nerve. Even if it is increasingly evident that several central neuroplastic mechanisms contribute to the pain, there are no studies suggesting that the somatotopic organization they induce is extensive enough to lead to false pain localization (see Chapters 7, 8, 12, 13, and 14). In many non-neuropathic unilateral conditions, typically referred pain from neck, atypical migraine, and giant cell arteritis, the patient describes a pain in trigeminal territory crossing into that of C2 or C3 roots.

Decision tree

If the answer is Yes, proceed to Question 3. If the answer is No, it is unlikely that the patient has cranial neuralgia or neuropathy, or TAC. Consider diagnostic options shown in the decision tree.

Question 3. Is the pain episodic?

True neuralgias and TACs share a temporal feature: the pain is episodic, with recurrent bouts that last from seconds to minutes and rarely beyond 1 hour. This time profile distinguishes them from continuous or near-continuous pain that defines painful neuropathies. We have noted that some patients struggle with the concept of timing and recommend that effort be made to clarify as well as possible. Expressions such as 'pain that comes and goes' or 'starts and stops suddenly' may help some patient to appreciate what is meant and focus on the issue. An occasional distressed patient may insist the pain is ever-present, perceived every second of every waking hour, only to admit they do not feel it the very moment of the interview. Diagrams may be used to elicit the pattern and timing (fig. 5.4).

An obvious caveat needing attention is combined episodic and continuous pain, experienced by many patients with TN and cluster headache (see Chapters 7, 12 and 14). If asked directly, most patients will be able identify which pain is more intense and hence the predominant feature. In true neuralgia, many will acknowledge that their background pain is not the one they want primarily abolished.

Decision tree

If the answer is Yes, proceed to Question 4. If the answer is No, proceed to establish whether or not there are sensory abnormalities in the affected area (Q3a

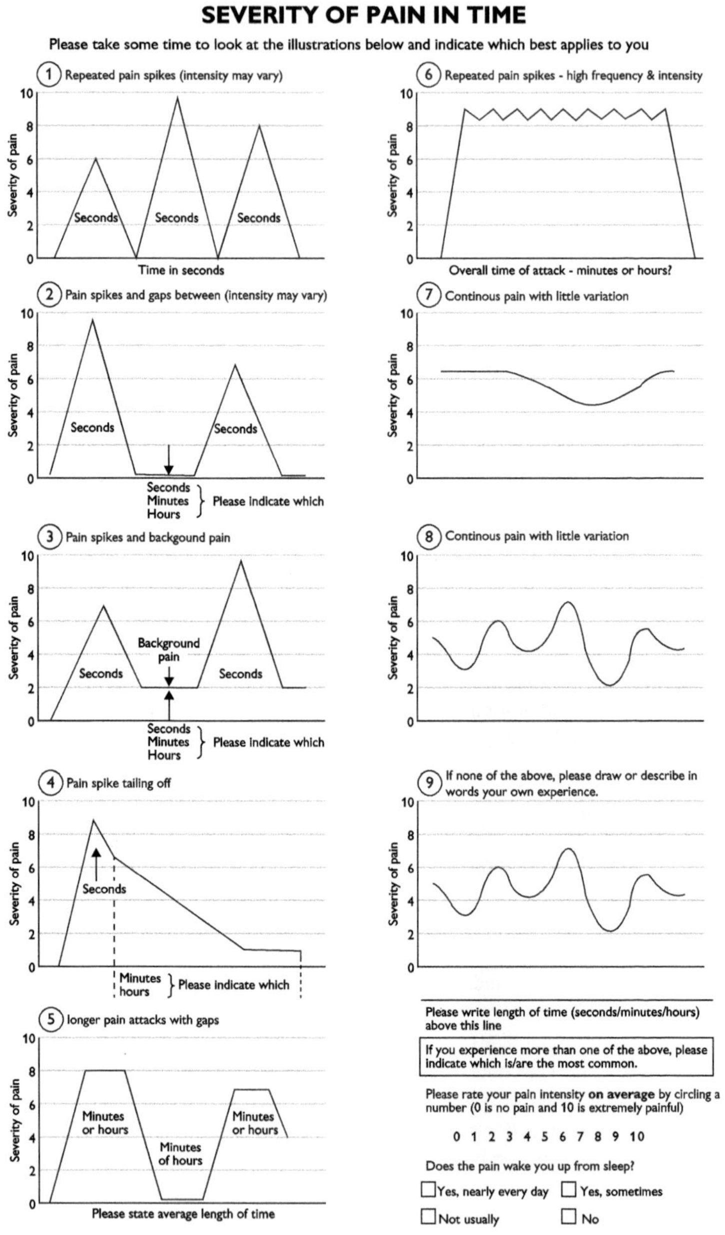

SEVERITY OF PAIN IN TIME

Please take some time to look at the illustrations below and indicate which best applies to you

(1) Repeated pain spikes (intensity may vary)

Severity of pain — 10, 8, 6, 4, 2, 0

Seconds / Seconds / Seconds

Time in seconds

(2) Pain spikes and gaps between (intensity may vary)

Severity of pain — 10, 8, 6, 4, 2, 0

Seconds / Seconds

Seconds / Minutes / Hours } Please indicate which

(3) Pain spikes and backgound pain

Severity of pain — 10, 8, 6, 4, 2, 0

Seconds / Background pain / Seconds

Seconds / Minutes / Hours } Please indicate which

(4) Pain spike tailing off

Severity of pain — 10, 8, 6, 4, 2, 0

Seconds

Minutes / hours } Please indicate which

(5) longer pain attacks with gaps

Severity of pain — 10, 8, 6, 4, 2, 0

Minutes or hours / Minutes of hours / Minutes or hours

Please state average length of time

(6) Repeated pain spikes - high frequency & intensity

Severity of pain — 10, 8, 6, 4, 2, 0

Overall time of attack - minutes or hours?

(7) Continous pain with little variation

Severity of pain — 10, 8, 6, 4, 2, 0

(8) Continous pain with little variation

Severity of pain — 10, 8, 6, 4, 2, 0

(9) If none of the above, please draw or describe in words your own experience.

Severity of pain — 10, 8, 6, 4, 2, 0

Please write length of time (seconds/minutes/hours) above this line

If you experience more than one of the above, please indicate which is/are the most common.

Please rate your pain intensity **on average** by circling a number (0 is no pain and 10 is extremely painful)

0 1 2 3 4 5 6 7 8 9 10

Does the pain wake you up from sleep?

☐ Yes, nearly every day ☐ Yes, sometimes

☐ Not usually ☐ No

Figure 5.4 Examples of types of temporal pain patterns

These can be discussed with patients and timing and severity inserted.

© A. Hale

in the algorithm). Any such abnormalities would define the condition as a painful neuropathy (see Chapter 11).

Question 4. Is the pain provoked by food rather than chewing or swallowing?

If the answer to the question is Yes, it is likely that the patient's pain is not due to a cranial neuralgia, neuropathy, or TAC, although there are several alternative diagnoses to entertain.

How the pain relates to eating is an important but tricky point to establish, if there is a connection that the patient has identified. It is helpful to try to focus on whether it is the act of eating, that is, chewing and swallowing, that provokes the pain. Generally speaking, pain associated with salivary gland stones (sialolithiasis) emerges slowly during a meal and continues well beyond it. Any food will induce the pain but spicy food in particular; the consistency of food plays little role. The pain is located on the floor of the mouth, an unusual site for cranial neuralgias. Palpation of the floor of the mouth may reveal a stone. Dental pulp disease will cause pain lasting seconds to minutes induced by hot and cold or sweet foods, and sometimes by lying supine. The hardest to distinguish is a cracked tooth as shown in fig. 5.5. The pain of a cracked tooth tends to occur on the rebound, that is, when the patient stops biting on the tooth, and will occur every time.

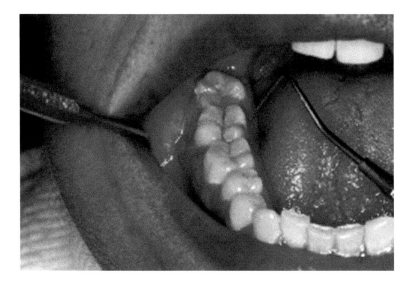

Figure 5.5 Cracked tooth
Note abscess, swelling, next to the second molar helps in the diagnosis.

Oral examination may reveal a tooth tender to percussion and caries and gingival swelling. In TN and glossopharyngeal neuralgia, the act of eating is what will provoke the pain, which usually appears abruptly at the beginning of the meal and in particular if the food requires strong chewing or effortful swallowing.

Pain which comes on after prolonged chewing, especially hard foods, and opening wide is mostly due to muscle pain from the masseter, lateral and medial pterygoids and relates to temporomandibular disorders. These can be unilateral and are very common especially in young people (see Chapter 15).

Decision tree

If eating does not provoke pain, or if pain is associated with the mechanics of eating only, proceed to Question 5.

Question 5. Are the pain episodes short lived (seconds to 2 minutes)?

The duration of any pain is of crucial significance in distinguishing cranial neuralgias from TACs. Attacks shorter than 2–3 minutes will strongly point toward TN while attacks of several minutes up to an hour suggest a TAC or another alterative atypical headache, such as atypical migraine or glaucoma. If the answer to Question 5 is No, then enquiring about the presence of autonomic symptoms during pain episodes allow one to determine if the pain is due to either cluster headache, paroxysmal hemicrania, or hemicrania continua (Question 5a). The quality and frequency of pain and presence of significant background pain will determine which of the three is in question. A detailed comparison is presented in Chapter 14 (see Table 14.1). Hemicrania continua presents with continuous pain interrupted with severe exacerbation lasting from half an hour to several hours; also much shorter bouts have been described. Cluster headache and paroxysmal hemicrania are not typically associated with continuous interictal pain.

Not all people are able to quantify the duration of their pain. One should consider offering examples with everyday time connotations, such as 'flash, stab, or jolt of pain'. We are wary about using the term 'electric shock' as most people have no personal experience of it, and some association with electricity in general is interpreted as a buzzing sensation. Auditory examples may work, too; one of the authors found a loud clap of hands to produce a similar startle reaction to the sudden pain that caught them unawares. However, in some patients with TN there is a very small gap between each attack.

The duration of individual pain attacks in short-lasting unilateral neuralgiform headache with conjunctival injection and tearing (SUNCT)/short-lasting unilateral neuralgiform headache with autonomic symptoms (SUNA) is similar to that in TN, so this question cannot distinguish the two.

A note on periodicity

Up to 50% of patients report the first episode as sudden and severe in onset and neurosurgeons have reported that patients with a memorable onset are more likely to have good outcomes after surgery. This first attack may be the most severe of all and hence memorable. A history of a refractory period (a post-paroxysm symptom-free couple of minutes during which mechanical stimuli do not trigger pain) is commonly elicited in patients with TN but not in those with SUNCT/SUNA.

Dental pain tends to come on gradually over days and weeks. Few chronic pain conditions result in remission periods and relapses and this can be a distinguishing feature from dental causes and trigeminal neuropathic pain.

Decision tree

If the answer to this question is Yes, proceed to Question 6.

If the answer is No, advance to Question 5a to explore details of pain attacks to establish whether the patient has cluster headache, paroxysmal hemicrania, or hemicrania continua.

Question 6. Is pain likely mediated by the trigeminal nerve? If not, which nerve is it in that case?

From the anatomical localization of pain and remembering that as per Question 2 it should be within a single nerve innervation territory. the interviewer will be able to deduce which nerve mediates the pain (trigeminal, glossopharyngeal, intermedius, auriculotemporal, superior laryngeal, and greater or lesser occipital nerve; see Chapters 6, 12, and 13).

Decision tree

For patients with pain in the trigeminal nerve territory go to Question 7. If not, you will have to decide on the nerve in question to arrive *at the final neuralgia diagnosis.*

Question 7. Are pain episodes associated with autonomic signs and symptoms?

Decision tree

If the answer is Yes: a strong positive history of ipsilateral autonomic symptoms and signs associated with individual pain attacks which include lacrimation, red eye, forehead sweating, runny or blocked nose, or facial flushing, *the likely final diagnosis is SUNCT or SUNA.* A negative history will leave TN and rare dental conditions (typically, cracked tooth or pulpitis). (Note: both TN and SUNA/SUNCT affecting the lower part of the face may be associated with mild autonomic symptoms, and careful questioning may be needed for differential diagnosis.)

If the answer is No, proceed to Question 8.

Question 8. Is there evidence of trigger zones? (Does the pain stop grooming?)

Any light-touch activities are likely to trigger a pain and patients will avoid washing, putting on makeup, and even grow beards to avoid shaving. Brushing the teeth is painful and plaque and a calculus can accumulate on the painful side as fig. 5.6 illustrates.

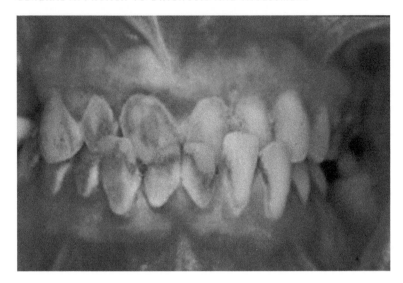

Figure 5.6 Poor oral hygiene on side of pain

A positive history should prompt an attempt to establish if the patient has any cutaneous or mucosal trigger zones (which are required for the diagnosis of TN, see Chapter 6). Clinical examination may not show any, and may not even be possible; however, almost without exception a reliable history can be elicited from those who have them.

The best method for separation of a tooth-related tenderness (cracked tooth) and a mucosal trigeminal trigger zone involves application of a gentle moving stimulus over the suspected site which in the case of TN will elicit a paroxysm. The path of radiation whether vertical or horizonal can be helpful in establishing the divisions that are involved.

This algorithm-based decision tree works as a general framework. In clinical practice, the final precision diagnosis requires exploring other clinical features with confirmatory questions, and an examination, before the final diagnosis is secured. Detailed clinical features are described in the relevant chapters.

5.4 Psychosocial assessment—the patient with the pain

Reaching the working diagnosis is the primary target of the first visit but alone insufficient for the management of the patient. The clinician must develop an understanding of the impact of the pain on the individual, how they respond to it, how it affects their physical and psychological functioning, and what consequences it has on the individual's social relationships. This extensive information cannot always be gathered during the first visit but can be supplemented at subsequent visits. On the initial visit, use of validated self-administered questionnaires is an effective way of extracting this information. Where regular follow-up visits are planned, they offer a convenient way of keeping track of the pain, treatment effects, and the patient's overall functioning. There are several validated questionnaires designed to cover various aspects of the pain experience, found suitable and recommended for neuropathic pain by an International Association for the Study of Pain Task Force but not all have been validated in TN.

Sleep has a significant impact on pain as it can both stop sleep or wake from sleep. A poor sleep pattern can also influence perception of pain.

5.4.1 Psychological assessment

A major factor that must be assessed in any patient with pain is its emotional and psychological impact. Anger, anxiety, and depression are common (see Chapter 16). Use of questionnaires before a visit will help the clinician to orient to any issues that may significantly impact management (Table 5.1). It is crucial to assess if there is a suicide risk as patients with TN and cluster headaches are known to commit suicide. Patients need to be asked if they perceive themselves to be at risk of suicide and this can be difficult to do. There are a variety of training aids available for this (e.g. see https://www.thriveldn.co.uk/campaigns/zerosuicideldn/).

5.4.2 Impact on activities of daily living

This should be determined and for that purpose there are several psychometrically tested questionnaires (Table 5.1). They can be used as outcome measures to ascertain the degree of overall pain management. Successful control of pain does not automatically mean that the patient's quality of life improves in parallel; for example, adverse effects of antineuralgic medication may drastically interfere with the patient's social functioning.

5.4.3 Social assessment

As for any patient, it is important to establish the home circumstances and support structures that are in place especially if surgery is planned. It is important to establish who the carer will be, who is at home with them, and what their relationships are. The patient may have other roles to perform which would impact their ability to manage their own facial pain. During severe episodes of pain, patients may be unable to work. If these are extended periods, they may even lose their jobs. This could be of significance especially if around retirement age and so could compromise their finances.

It is important to establish that the patient has a good grasp of the language in which the consultation is carried out. If this is poor than an approved interpreter is required as family members and friends may introduce bias into the consultation.

Table 5.1 Recommended psychometric questionnaires for facial pain patients		
Category	Measurement tool	Data collection
Intensity of pain*	Numerical rating scale, NRS (0–10) Visual analogue scale, VAS (0–100 or 0–10)	On all visits and contacts
Affect*	Beck Depression Inventory, BDI-II Hospital Anxiety and Depression Scale, HADS Profile of Mood States, POMS	At onset/during treatment if needed/at end of treatment
Catastrophizing	Pain Catastrophizing Scale, PCS	At onset and end of treatment
Impact on daily living/ interference*	Brief Pain Inventory, BPI Work Productivity and Activity Impairment Questionnaire, WPAI	At onset/during treatment if needed/at end of treatment
Quality of life*	EQ-5D-5L WHO Quality of Life Questionnaire, WHOQOL	At onset and end of treatment
Treatment effect	Patient Global Impression of Change, PGIC	At end of treatment
Treatment Satisfaction	Treatment Satisfaction Scale	At end of treatment
For specialist clinic use		
General impact— cluster headache	Headache Impact Test, HIT-6	At onset and end of treatment
Quality of life— cluster headache/TN	Cluster Headache Quality of Life Scale, CHQ**/Trigeminal Neuralgia QoL Scale, TNQOLS**	At onset and end of treatment
Treatment effects—neurosurgery	Barlow Neurological Institute pain score, BNI**	At end of treatment
Interference in daily activities	Penn Facial Pain Scale Revised, PENN-FPS-R**	At onset and end of treatment

*Essential category to measure (use one measure only) **Additional validation needed.
Details of data collection and assessment available from the Faculty of Pain Medicine website: https://fpm.ac.uk/sites/fpm/files/documents/2019-07/Outcome%20measures%202019.pdf
Source data from Nova CV, Zakrzewska JM, Baker SR, Riordain RN. Treatment Outcomes in Trigeminal Neuralgia-A Systematic Review of Domains, Dimensions and Measures. World Neurosurg X. 2020 Jan 27;6:100070. doi: 10.1016/j.wnsx.2020.100070. Accessed on 22/01/2022

Determining their social and leisure interests or activities can be important in establishing outcomes that they want to achieve (e.g. singing, gardening). Social isolation is very common among patients whose pain is provoked by eating as many social events centre on food.

CHAPTER 5

Box 5.1 Embedded in this case scenario are answers to the eight questions of the training tool. What is the diagnosis?

TD female 46 years old.

Pain first started: early 2011, while dining in a restaurant.

Preceding event: nil

Severity of pain on a scale of 0–10. Average 5, worst 8, least 3. More severe each time it recurs.

Timing: first episode lasted a few weeks, recurred April 2012 for a few weeks but then restarted July 2012. Episodic paroxysms last for a few seconds. They start suddenly and resolve suddenly and there is a remission period of hours in between attacks.

Character: sharp, prickling, shooting, pinching, tingling, frightful and tight.

Location: always right-sided cheek and lower jaw, can be felt intra- and extraoral.

Factors affecting pain: provoked by eating, chewing, irrespective of the type of food, does not continue beyond eating. Sometimes provoked by brushing her teeth, washing face. Stress and tension can aggravate her episodes.

Associated factors:

1. No eye, ear, nose symptoms.
2. Sleep not affected.
3. No other chronic pain, no headaches or migraines.

Social and family history: pharmacy assistant but lost her job mainly due to taking time off and sick leave due to her pain.

A family history of cranial neuralgias should be established. Although most cases are sporadic, a small percentage turn out to be familial, and this has been observed with most neuralgias, in particular cluster headache and TN.

Please take a moment to read the patient study in Box 5.1; what is the probable diagnosis?

5.5 Clinical examination

When the history strongly points to a particular diagnosis, there is a temptation to skip any examination but such temptation such be resisted. In practically all situations somatosensory examination is necessary, and should include tests for sharpness and light touch, as well as mechanical allodynia. Simple 'bedside' tests are generally sufficient. (Some may prefer more sophisticated quantitative sensory testing if the method is readily available.) When involvement of the trigeminal nerve is suspected, all three divisions are tested bilaterally. Sensory testing of the glossopharyngeal nerve is difficult but can be replaced by testing the gag reflex. Occipital nerves are tested on both sides. The main purpose for the sensory examination is to distinguish between pain conditions and look for major neural pathology behind the symptoms. Even when the history is entirely compatible with TN, one cannot know whether it is secondary to a tumour or multiple sclerosis; such patients, however, commonly show sensory abnormalities and other neurological signs even if subtle. Somatosensory examination is needed to confirm cranial nerve dysfunction which is the hallmark sign of cranial mononeuropathies. It is important to appreciate the difference pain evoked by gently tapping on a very small skin (trigger zone) from that evoked by moving a brush across a larger skin area (dynamic mechanical allodynia). The former is seen in TN and the latter in trigeminal neuropathy.

Intraoral examination is equally important with attention paid to the level of oral hygiene, status of the gingiva, and any tooth tenderness to percussion. Even in the case of a straightforward TN, a tooth problem may act as a trigger. Evidence of frictional keratosis in the buccal mucosa will provide evidence of clenching (fig. 5.7). Testing of muscle function, such as jaw opening and neck movements, and tenderness of masticatory muscles helps to complete the picture. A systematic assessment of all cranial nerves is rarely of use. It is best left for occasions when there are other neurological signs independent of pain, such as unsteadiness of gait, slurred speech, or ophthalmoplegia.

Once the history and examination has been completed, a discussion has taken place, and a patient-centred treatment plan determined, a careful record needs to be made. Record keeping is essential as the stories can change as patients reflect

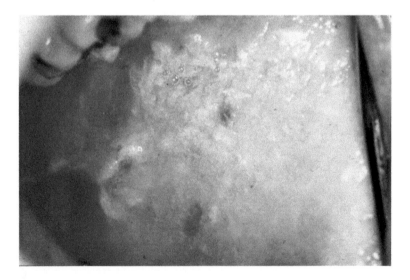

Figure 5.7 Frictional keratosis
May be only a linear line along the occlusal line or more extensive chewing of the whole cheek.

on their pain episodes in the light of the interview. Pain diaries can be helpful as prompts as patients will often only remember their worse periods and yet the length of remission and relapse periods is important to try to establish whether there is progression with time. Use of standard psychometric questionnaires is the most reliable way of keeping track of the effectiveness and safety of the management of the pain (Table 5.1). All this material will be very useful for any clinical audit.

5.6 Investigations

5.6.1 Imaging

TN, the most common type of cranial neuralgia, is currently identified by its clinical presentation as there are no specific tests—imaging or otherwise—that can be considered diagnostic of this condition. Nonetheless, the wealth of clinical and surgical experience strongly supports the role of imaging in helping precision diagnosis, to establish the aetiology when specific clinical criteria are met. For example, imaging can identify the presence of neurovascular compression (NVC) as a key feature of TN. Identification of NVC is important because it can help classify the type of trigeminal pain (under International Classification of Headache Disorders, third edition (ICDH-3) criteria, see Chapter 6). This will then help the clinician in their treatment decision-making.

The presence of NVC is defined as proximity and contact between a vascular structure and the trigeminal nerve. This is seen most commonly at the trigeminal root entry zone. The type of compression can vary, consisting of contact, compression, or frank distortion (fig. 5.8).

An important clinical point should be noted that the type of compression does not, however, correlate with severity of TN pain. While ICDH-3 criteria distinguish subtypes of TN based on the presence of NVC (such as classical and idiopathic types), the clinical expression of pain in these syndromes can be identical. Thus, many research groups, including ours, are beginning to shift their focus from the study of the vascular compression to studies of the trigeminal nerve itself and how structural nerve abnormalities in TN can correlate with the expression of pain.

Magnetic resonance imaging

NVC is best visualized on axial magnetic resonance images acquired with thin cut sequences such as fast imaging employing steady-state acquisition (FIESTA), three-dimensional (3D) constructive interference in steady state (CISS), or other similar sequences. These images should be performed in sufficiently thin cuts (1 mm, no gap) to visualize the root entry zone and course of the trigeminal nerve, and surrounding vasculature (fig. 5.9). Although coronal images can demonstrate NVC, they may not be part of the clinical practice or routinely acquired. A similar technique can be used to look for NVC of the glossopharyngeal nerve or facial-vestibular nerve complex in the context of other neuralgias (see Chapter 12).

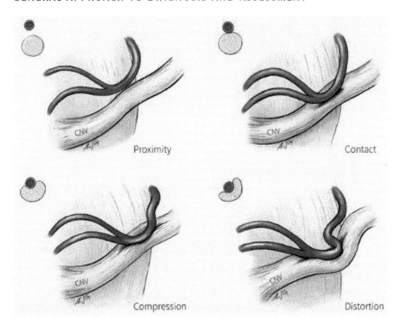

Figure 5.8 Types of neurovascular compression

Types of neurovascular conflict.

Reproduced from DeSouza DD, Hodaie M, Davis KD. Structural magnetic resonance imaging can identify trigeminal system abnormalities in classical trigeminal neuralgia. Front Neuroanat. 2016 Oct 19;10:95. doi.org/10.3389/fnana.2016.00095, under CC BY

Two other magnetic resonance sequences are highly informative. A T2-weighted or FLAIR sequence through the whole head can help identify possible pathology that points to multiple sclerosis. Full head, thin cut T1-weighted images have also proved invaluable to identify a newly described syndrome of TN that is associated with a single pontine lesion (SPL-TN) (fig. 5.10). It is important to identify this unusual syndrome to inform treatment plans because these patients rarely show good long-term response to surgical treatment or may often—incorrectly—be diagnosed with multiple sclerosis. Based on our recent study describing this entity, their rate is 5%.

The role of a routine 'screening' MRI

Investigation of a newly diagnosed patient with TN frequently leads to a routine 'screening' MRI study. This type of imaging generally has limited value, as the visualization of the root of the trigeminal nerve may be limited, subsequently resulting in limited visualization of possible NVC. Screening MRIs may be done in thicker slices (3–5 mm) which, while helpful in demonstrating large scale abnormalities,

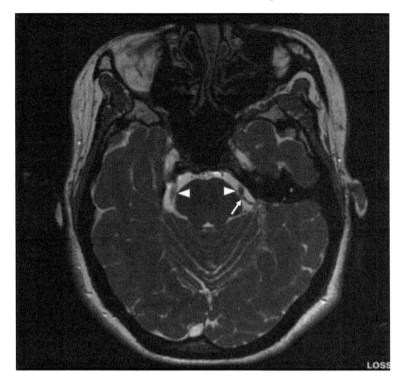

Figure 5.9 Axial FIESTA images—trigeminal nerve

FIESTA images showing the anatomical course of the trigeminal nerve through the cisternal space. Neurovascular contact at the left root entry zone can be visualized.

may in turn show little anatomical detail of the trigeminal nerve. It is also very important for the clinician to develop the practice of evaluating the MRIs. Frequently MRIs are reported as 'normal' given that no specific anatomical abnormality exists (for instance, there is no tumour or demyelination). It is therefore imperative to provide specific comments on the MRI request to allow the radiologist to adequately investigate this crucial anatomical detail.

Upon visualizing the nerve, the position of the root entry zone, possible kinking/distortion, as well as a qualitative assessment of the volume of the nerve should be documented. Furthermore, it should be noted whether there is possible atrophy and vascular structures that would primarily impinge the root entry zone and less commonly, further distally. This information has utility because the root entry zone is characterized by the interface of central versus peripheral myelin. This interface is chiefly conical in shape and may protrude inside the presumed cisternal segment by at least several millimetres. It is believed that

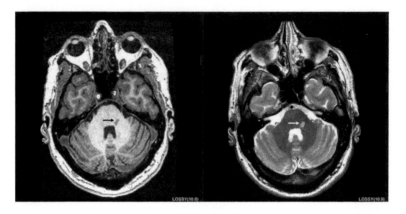

Figure 5.10 Single pontine lesion

Axial FSPGR and axial T2-weighted images through the area of the pons in a patient with single-pontine-lesion TN. The lesion affects the brainstem fibres of the trigeminal nerve. The cisternal fibres are otherwise unaffected.

compression over this potential weak area is chiefly responsible for the possible areas of focal demyelination that are observed upon pathological examination of TN nerves, as described by Love and Coakham (2000). It is therefore fitting that most instances of NVC are observed at the root entry zone and less commonly, further distally.

A patient's MRIs should be examined to identify the type of compression, whether arterial or venous. Arterial compression is significantly more common than venous NVC. It is not uncommon to observe both an artery and a vein compressing the vessel although at times this is observed with greater clarity during a microvascular decompression procedure. Lastly, for the purposes of planning the decompression procedure, the degree of compression should be evaluated to determine whether the vascular structure is simply approaching the nerve, compressing it, or frankly distorting it. The most extreme type of distortion of the nerve is in the setting of dolichoectatic basilar arteries where the large structure of the basilar artery can significantly distort that nerve.

Other anatomical causes of trigeminal compression

The nerve may not only be compressed by a vessel but also by arachnoidal bands that may compress the root of the nerve. A thick band of arachnoid generally holds the superior petrosal vein, and this band often needs to be divided during microvascular decompression, to allow for adequate visualization of the nerve. The anatomy of the root entry zone allows for great interindividual variability in skull base anatomy, and particularly the distance between the petrosal vein entry into the petrosal sinus and the root of the trigeminal nerve. This implies that some arachnoidal bands may also hold the trigeminal nerve. This is often difficult to see on MRI. For this reason, patients with idiopathic TN may also be surgical candidates and undergo successful microvascular decompression.

The presence of bilateral NVC

Several studies, dating back to Miller et al. (2009) have addressed the role of NVC in TN and compared its presence in a healthy population. It is rather surprising, but notable, that the presence of bilateral NVC has been observed in TN, in a much greater proportion than in the non-TN population (see 'Recommended reading'). Nearly 40% of patients with TN show bilateral NVC, even though the pain is uniformly unilateral (fig. 5.11). In a comparable healthy control population, less than 20% have evidence of NVC. At the same time, over 35% of patients with a clinical diagnosis of TN do not show any evidence of vascular compression.

Diffusion tensor imaging (DTI) can be used to quantify microstructural metrics (see 'Recommended reading') and has demonstrated that there are microstructural abnormalities in the root entry zone of symptomatic TN nerves. Interestingly, DTI also demonstrated significant bilateral differences in the trigeminal root entry zone, though there was a much more notable difference between the trigeminal nerves in a healthy population and nerves symptomatic for TN. These findings are in concordance with the findings of Miller and colleagues.

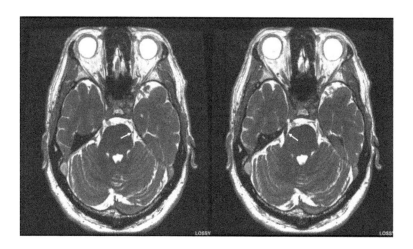

Figure 5.11 Axial FIESTA—bilateral neurovascular compression

FIESTA images of patient with TN, demonstrating neurovascular contact bilaterally at the root entry zone of the trigeminal nerve. The patient is symptomatic with severe left-sided pain.

CHAPTER 5

The role of DTI in the study of TN

The addition of DTI provides a novel approach to study TN with great potential utility for clinical diagnostics and treatment planning (fig. 5.12).

DTI is sensitive to water anisotropy—the preferential movement of water in specific directions along the nerve fibres. This implies that DTI can differentiate the microstructural environment, to inform on TN-specific abnormalities. Though not yet part of the routine imaging of patients with TN, over the past decade DTI studies of TN abnormalities have transformed the field and introduced the valuable role of an *in vivo* technique that may serve to assess and distinguish this syndrome, as well as the effect of treatment on the nerve. Key work in this area has pointed to microstructural diffusion metrics that distinguish surgical treatment responders from non-responders. Examination of the pre-treatment MRI in TN demonstrates that individuals who go on to achieve long-term pain-free status after surgical treatment have abnormal diffusion metrics that focus on the root entry zone or cisternal component of the nerve (Hung et al., 2017) whereas eventual non-responders have altered metrics in the brainstem fibres

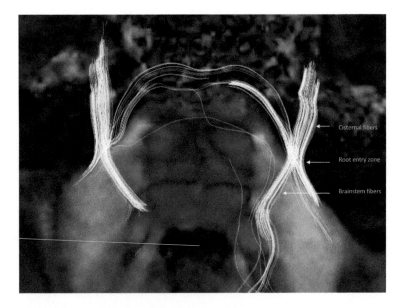

Figure 5.12 DTI of the trigeminal nerves

DTI of the trigeminal nerves using extended streamline tractography, demonstrating the position of the root entry zone, cisternal fibres, and importantly, the brainstem fibres of the trigeminal nerve.

Reproduced from Tohyama S, et al. Trigeminal neuralgia associated with a solitary pontine lesion: clinical and neuroimaging definition of a new syndrome. Pain. 2020 May;161(5):916–925. doi: 10.1097/j.pain.0000000000001777 with permission from Wolters Kluwer Health, Inc

of the trigeminal nerve. This suggests that despite a similar expression of pain in responders and non-responders, these two groups may be distinguished based on their microstructural features. Further study of this area will help the use of these novel imaging modalities as a tool to guide treatment and counsel patients. DTI may also shed light on the likelihood of response to treatment. Gamma Knife radiosurgery is a common form of treatment of TN consisting of delivery of a sharp beam of radiation to the nerve. Conventional MRI is not able to pinpoint tools that can define the clinical outcome of radiosurgery. DTI, however, demonstrates a drop in fractional anisotropy of the trigeminal nerve in those who will be long-term responders to treatment and no significant drop in fractional anisotropy in non-responders.

While imaging is not diagnostic of TN, it has always been an important adjunct, particularly in the identification of NVC. Newer imaging modalities including DTI have helped identify new TN subtypes such as SPL-TN. Importantly, newer imaging modalities may lead to advances which will increase the value of imaging, distinguish between subtypes, and provide better guidance for treatment.

5.6.2 Neurophysiological testing

Neurophysiological investigations help to distinguish patients with primary (i.e. classical and idiopathic) and secondary TN. Neurophysiological investigation in patients with TN mainly include trigeminal reflex tests and nociceptive evoked potentials.

Trigeminal reflex tests

Trigeminal reflex recording is the most useful and reliable neurophysiological procedure for investigating trigeminal system. Trigeminal reflexes consist of different reflex responses, including the blink reflex and the masseter inhibitory reflex. These two reflex responses assess the function of large myelinated non-nociceptive trigeminal afferents from all trigeminal territories, as well as their trigeminal central circuits in the pons and medulla.

The *blink reflex* evoked by electrical stimulation of the supraorbital nerve comprises two responses. The first, R1, not clinically visible, occurs at a 10 ms latency ipsilateral to the side of the stimulation. The second, R2, has a 30 ms latency, is bilateral, and more prolonged. The afferent impulses for the R1 are relayed through a short oligosynaptic circuit to the facial motoneurons. Nerve impulses responsible for R2 are conducted through the spinal tract in the dorsolateral region of the pons and medulla before they reach the spinal trigeminal nucleus. From there, impulses are further relayed to a polysynaptic chain of reticular interneurons; the last interneuron sends ipsilateral and contralateral collaterals that ascend to the facial nuclei in the lower pons (fig. 5.13).

Electrical stimulation of the infraorbital and mental nerve evokes a reflex inhibition of the jaw-closing muscles, the *masseter inhibitory reflex*. This reflex inhibition consists of an early and a late silent period, SP1 and SP2. The SP1 response is probably mediated by one inhibitory interneuron, located close to the ipsilateral

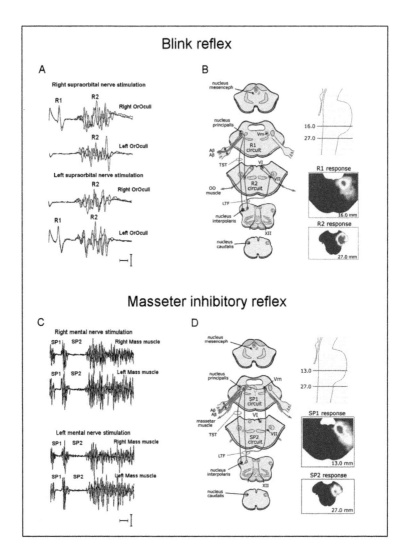

Figure 5.13 Blink and masseter inhibitory reflexes

Normal blink reflex (A) and masseter inhibitory reflex (C) recordings. Surface recordings from the right and left relaxed orbicularis oculi muscles (OO muscles) and contracted masseter muscles (Mass muscles). Superimposed trials in a healthy subject. Electrical stimulation of the supraorbital nerve elicits an ipsilateral R1 response and a bilateral R2 response. Electrical stimulation of the mental nerve elicits SP1 and SP2 responses (silent periods) bilaterally. Calibration 10 ms/200 µV in A and 20 ms/100 µV in C.

Blink reflex and masseter inhibitory reflex circuits (B and D). Large myelinated (Aβ) primary afferents from the ophthalmic division enter the pons. Impulses for the R1 are conveyed to the ipsilateral orbicularis oculi (OO) motoneurons in the facial nucleus (VII). Afferents for R2 descend in the trigeminospinal tract (TST) to the medulla; in the nucleus interpolaris they connect with a polysynaptic chain of excitatory interneurons of the lateral reticular formation; the last interneuron sends ipsi- and contralateral axons that ascend through the lateral tegmental field (LTF) to reach the OO motoneurons bilaterally.

Reproduced from Cruccu G, Iannetti GD, Truini A. Brainstem reflexes and their relevance to pain. Handb Clin Neurol. 2006;81:411–IX. doi: 10.1016/S0072-9752(06)80032-1 with permission from Elsevier.

trigeminal motor nucleus. The SP2 circuit includes a polysynaptic chain descending to the spinal trigeminal nucleus, pars interpolaris. The last interneuron of the chain is inhibitory and gives rise to ipsilateral and contralateral collaterals ascending to reach the jaw-closing motoneurons in the masticatory nuclei (fig. 5.13).

Trigeminal reflex testing is particularly useful in patients who cannot undergo MRI, or to demonstrate demyelination and disclose trigeminal neuropathies mimicking classical TN. A diagnostic protocol for patients with trigeminal pain should rely primarily on trigeminal reflex tests: the finding of any abnormality implies an underlying structural lesion. Abnormalities are often disclosed in divisions that appear clinically unaffected. In secondary TN, trigeminal reflexes invariably show abnormalities. Concordant studies showed that trigeminal reflex tests are sensitive and specific for diagnosing secondary TN. Current guidelines on TN management report that trigeminal reflex testing has high sensitivity and specificity in diagnosing secondary TN (88% and 94%). Posterior fossa tumours producing mechanical damage to the proximal portion of the trigeminal root or a demyelinating plaque affecting the intrapontine presynaptic primary afferents near the root entry zone typically produce abnormalities of all responses (fig. 5.14).

Nociceptive evoked potentials

The easiest and most reliable neurophysiological techniques for assessing nociceptive pathway function are laser-evoked potentials and contact heat-evoked potentials. Using laser radiant or contact heating the two techniques selectively activate Aδ and C nociceptors in the most superficial skin layers and evoked scalp potentials consisting of a lateralized component N1, generated by opercular parietal region and a large-amplitude vertex complex, N2–P2, generated by anterior insular and cingulate cortices (fig. 5.15 and fig. 5.16). Contrary to what was believed in the past, recordings using surface concentric electrodes are not suitable for investigating nociceptive pathways.

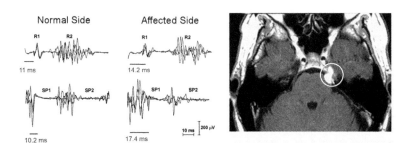

Figure 5.14 Blink reflex and masseter inhibitory reflex recording in a patient with TN due to a posterior fossa tumour

The latency delay of R1 and SP1 responses after stimulation of the affected side.

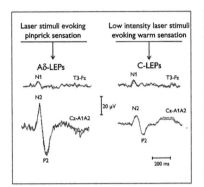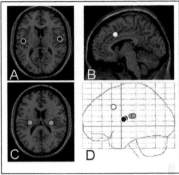

Figure 5.15 Laser-evoked potentials

Left panel: laser-evoked potentials related to the activation of Aδ and C fibres after stimulation of the perioral regions. Relatively high-intensity laser stimulation evokes pinprick sensation and Aδ fibre-related laser-evoked potentials; low-intensity laser stimulation activates thermal C-receptors and elicit C-fibre-related laser-evoked potentials.

Right panel: generators of laser-evoked potentials. (A,C) Axial sections showing the generators of the early negativity (N1), localized bilaterally in the parietal operculum (black dots) and insula (gray dots). (B) Sagittal section showing the generator of the main N2–P2 complex in the posterior part of the anterior cingulate gyrus (white dot). (D) Glass brain showing all dipoles in lateral view.

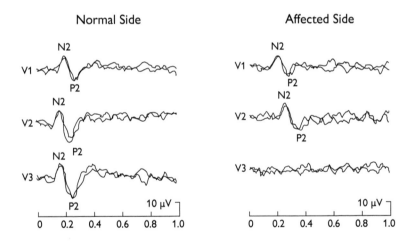

Figure 5.16 Laser-evoked potentials in a patient with classical TN

Two series of ten artefact-free trials collected and averaged after stimulation of the supraorbital (V1), upper lip (V2), and lower lip skin (V3) on the right and left sides. Recordings from the vertex referenced to linked earlobes. Note the delay (V2) or absence (V3) of the laser-evoked potential after stimulation of the affected territory.

Adapted from Cruccu G, Leandri M, Iannetti GD, Mascia A, Romaniello A, Truini A, Galeotti F, Manfredi M. Small-fiber dysfunction in trigeminal neuralgia: carbamazepine effect on laser-evoked potentials. Neurology. 2001 Jun 26;56(12):1722–6. doi: 10.1212/wnl.56.12.1722 with permission from Wolters Kluwer Health, Inc.

The trigeminal territory is particularly advantageous for laser and contact heat-evoked potential recording because of the short conduction distance that minimizes the problem of signal dispersion along slow-conducting unmyelinated afferents, and the high receptor density. Nociceptive evoked potentials related to Aδ and C fibres are of higher amplitude and are recorded more easily than those after limb stimulation.

However, currently laser-evoked and contact heat-evoked potentials have a limited usefulness in the differential diagnosis of classical and idiopathic forms from secondary TN because of poor specificity. They may be better suited to investigate the integrity of small myelinated and unmyelinated fibres in patients with other neuropathic facial pain conditions, including rare trigeminal isolated sensory neuropathies.

5.7 Lay summaries

5.7.1 Lay summary: history and assessment

Patients need to provide a comprehensive history of their facial pain as there are no other ways of making a diagnosis. A series of specific questions have been established which help to make a diagnosis of TN. Questionnaires are added tools that can be used by healthcare professionals to especially assess the impact of pain on activities of daily living and on mood. Knowing more about a patient's social life can help doctors to tailor treatment plans more specifically.

5.7.2 Lay summary: investigations

MRI is the principal method for investigating the cause of trigeminal and other cranial neuralgias. An MRI scan is performed after the doctor has determined from the patient's symptoms that they suffer from a neuralgia pain.

When specific MRI techniques are employed, the scan will identify any structure compressing the nerve to make it painful. This can be a blood vessel, a tumour, or a band of brain membrane. The scan is also useful in showing if the pain is due to a disease, such as multiple sclerosis affecting brain pain pathways in a way that makes them generate pain attacks.

A new research technique, DTI, is designed to track bundles of nerve fibres and reveal signs of damage to them and may help neurosurgeons in the future to decide the suitability of the patient for a procedure.

Neurophysiological tests are useful when the patient cannot have an MRI scan. Trigeminal brainstem reflexes help to decide if the neuralgia is caused by multiple sclerosis or a tumour but they do not tell if the nerve is compressed by a blood vessel or not.

5.8 RECOMMENDED READING

Cruccu G, Iannetti GD, Truini A. Chapter 28. Brainstem reflexes and their relevance to pain. Handb Clin Neurol. 2006;81:411–IX. doi: 10.1016/S0072-9752(06)80032-1

DeSouza DD, Hodaie M, Davis KD. Structural magnetic resonance imaging can identify trigeminal system abnormalities in classical trigeminal neuralgia. Front Neuroanat. 2016;10:95. doi: 10.3389/fnana.2016.00095

Hung PS, Chen DQ, Davis KD, et al. Predicting pain relief: use of pre-surgical trigeminal nerve diffusion metrics in trigeminal neuralgia. Neuroimage Clin. 2017;15:710–8. doi: 10.1016/j.nicl.2017.06.017

Love S, Coakham HB. Trigeminal neuralgia: pathology and pathogenesis. Brain. 2001;124:2347–60. doi: 10.1093/brain/124.12.2347

Miller JP, Acar F, Hamilton BE, et al. Radiographic evaluation of trigeminal neurovascular compression in patients with and without trigeminal neuralgia. J Neurosurg. 2009;110:627–32. doi: 10.3171/2008.6.17620

Tohyama S, Hung PS, Cheng JC, et al. Trigeminal neuralgia associated with a solitary pontine lesion: clinical and neuroimaging definition of a new syndrome. Pain. 2020;161:916–25. doi: 10.1097/j.pain.0000000000001777

Ziegeler C, May A. Facial presentations of migraine, TACs, and other paroxysmal facial pain syndromes. Neurology 2019;93:e1138–47. doi: 10.1212/WNL.0000000000008124

5.9 Continuing professional development

History and assessment

1. A patient presents with pain in the lower part of the face. Which statements will help to distinguish between TN and other facial pain True/false:
   a. Continuous pain with flare ups. T/F
   b. Episodic pain with each episode of pain lasting 30 minutes T/F
   c. Always on the same side of the face in a nerve distribution T/F
   d. Provoked by prolonged eating T/F
   e. Can be associated with ipsilateral red eye and tearing. T/F
2. List four reasons why a family and social history are important.
3. Patient reports a sharp pain when a piece of cotton wool is moved across the left cheek. What is your working diagnosis and what else would you expect the clinical examination show?
4. Name at least two questionnaires suitable for determining depression in a patient with cranial neuralgia.
5. What is the diagnosis of the patient in Box 5.1? (You can use the diagnostic training tool).
6. The patient scenario in Box 5.2 (see below) provides a history and results of questionnaires—what does it tell you and how is it going to affect your treatment plan?

Investigations

7. Explain why routine MRI is not the optimal method for investigating a patient with TN.

8. On reviewing an MRI scan of a patient with TN, which anatomical structures should you focus on and why? What changes will you be looking for?

9. What is the potential advantage of use of DTI in the evaluation of TN?

10. Name and briefly describe the two trigeminal reflex tests.

Box 5.2 Patient scenario (Question 6)

Female patient aged 56 years old has had pain on and off for the last 6 years. She works as a personal assistant to a finance officer and has had to take more than a month off work in the last 6 months. She is married and her husband is semi-retired and their son still lives with them.

Results of psychometrically tested questionnaires:

Brief Pain Inventory: mean pain intensity 7.5 (range 0–10), impact on seven activities of daily living 8.1 (range 0–10), impact on seven facial activities 9.7 (range 0–10).

Hospital Anxiety and Depression Scale: Anxiety 13, Depression 14; scores above 11 are significant.

Pain Catastrophising Scale: score 36; scores above 24 considered significant.

Trigeminal neuralgia: Diagnosis and classification

Turo Nurmikko and Joanna M. Zakrzewska

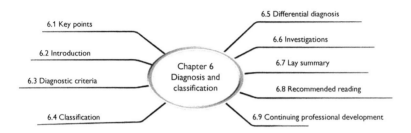

Figure 6.1 Plan of chapter

6.1 KEY POINTS

1. Trigeminal neuralgia is diagnosed clinically, on the basis of quality of pain (severe, short-lived paroxysms), location (unilateral, trigeminal territory), and provocative factors (innocuous mechanical stimuli).

2. It is divided into three aetiological subcategories: classical (with magnetic resonance imaging evidence of significant neurovascular compression), idiopathic (no significant compression or other cause), and symptomatic (with other cause identified, e.g. tumour, multiple sclerosis).

3. All three subcategories include patients presenting with one of two different phenotypes: paroxysmal only and with concomitant continuous pain.

4. Important differential diagnoses include short-lasting unilateral neuralgiform headache with conjunctival injection and tearing (SUNCT)/short-lasting unilateral neuralgiform headache with autonomic symptoms (SUNA) (see Chapter 14), trigeminal neuropathy (see Chapter 11), persistent idiopathic facial pain (see Chapter 15), and temporomandibular disorders (see Chapter 15).

6.2 Introduction

Although at first glance it would appear that trigeminal neuralgia (TN) is easy to diagnose and there are clear criteria, over the years this has proven to be a complex diagnosis and many caveats are used when describing it. Other names that have been used include tic douloureux, atypical TN, and TN type 1 or 2.

As we have seen in Chapter 2, there have been a variety of classifications put forward by different organizations and an attempt has been made to operationalize these. The new classifications have led to better harmonization of research studies and clinical databases which may now be more comparable. The addition of notes and comments especially in the International Classification of Headache Disorders, third edition (ICHD-3) and the first edition of the International Classification of Orofacial Pain (ICOP-1) criteria allow for improved diagnosis to be made in the clinical setting.

6.3 Diagnostic criteria: ICHD-3 and ICOP-1

The pain has all the following characteristics:

A. Recurrent paroxysms of unilateral facial pain in the distribution(s) of one or more divisions of the trigeminal nerve, with no radiation beyond, and fulfilling criteria B and C.

B. Pain has all of the following characteristics:
    1. Lasting from a fraction of a second to 2 minutes.
    2. Severe intensity.
    3. Electric shock-like, shooting, stabbing, or sharp in quality.

C. Precipitated by innocuous stimuli within the affected trigeminal distribution.

D. Not better accounted for by another diagnosis.

It is recognized that changes can occur over time especially in that attacks are:

- More intense.
- Longer.
- Not all evoked, some spontaneous.

Patients will often report a memorable onset, that is, they remember what they were doing when they experienced their first attack of pain. Some patients will report a refractory period but this can be difficult to elicit. Witnessing an attack which results in pain-induced facial muscle twitches is highly characteristic. These muscle spasms, if frequent, could lead to background pain. As movement and touching the face results in pain, patients will keep still during attacks, avoid brushing their teeth, eat very soft food, and avoid going out in cold wind. It can result in weight loss. For further impacts of TN on quality of life, (see Chapters 16, 17, and 19).

6.4 Classification of trigeminal neuralgia

Based on aetiology, three major subtypes of TN are distinguished (ICHD-3, ICOP-1):

1. Classical TN:
   - Neurovascular compression demonstrated on magnetic resonance imaging (MRI) or during operation of neurovascular compression causing root atrophy or displacement.

2. Idiopathic TN:
   • No significant compression (simple contact not causing changes in nerve root allowed).
3. Secondary TN:
   • An underlying cause, other than vascular compression, has been demonstrated.

Concomitant continuous pain may be associated with all three subtypes.

A careful history, clinical examination, and investigations as discussed in Chapter 5 allow for the TN subtypes to be recognized as summarized in fig. 6.2. More details are given in Chapters 7 and 8.

6.5 Differential diagnosis

The two patient scenarios in Table 6.1 demonstrate the key features that need to be addressed for a complete assessment of a patient with suspected TN.

There are a few case descriptions in the literature of a condition which has been termed pre-TN in which the patient initially reports a more nondescript pain which later becomes a classical TN.

It has been suggested in some descriptions of persistent idiopathic facial pain (PIFP) that it could be related to trauma but according to the new classification it

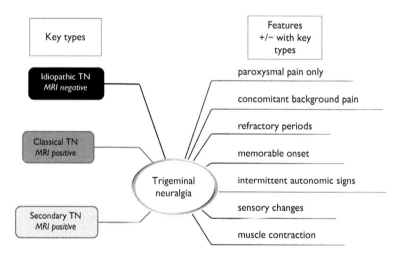

Figure 6.2 Summary of TN subcategories

The three subcategories are shown on the left and each of these will have one or more features listed on the right.

Table 6.1 Two patient scenarios

Features	Patient 1	Patient 2
Sex, age	Female, 52 years	Female, 54 years
History of pain	10 years ago possible toothache, root canal therapy, and no pain for 2 years, since then regular periods of pain and phenotype not changed	First attack of TN in 2006, gradually more severe, microvascular decompression in 2008, pain free for 9 years. Since 2017 on and off medication but pain has gradually been increasing in severity but not as severe as preoperatively
Character/quality	Stabbing, shooting, residual throbbing, nagging, burning	Not shooting electric quality, feels like a spasm, wrenching, aching, heavy but sharp pain at times
Site and radiation	Unilateral right centred over the cheek and felt in the upper teeth	Same location right side, starts inside ear, and then radiates down whole of V3 area
Severity on visual analogue scale, 0–10 cm	7–10/10	3–4/10
Duration and periodicity	Sudden onset, severe for a few seconds followed by a milder pain lasting 1 hour, burning discomfort for hours. Severe attacks sometimes every 30 minutes but on average 5 a day. Relapses of 2–3 weeks, remission periods of 2–3 months	Attacks of seconds can be every 10 min but remains with background aching pain most of the time
Provoking factors	Eating, brushing teeth, touching cheek, cold wind, flying	Eating, brushing teeth, cold
Relieving factors	Nil	Low-dose oxcarbazepine
Associated factors	Intermittent headaches, mild migraines with no aura 1–2 times per month, neck pain, no autonomic features	Migraine with aura, sumatriptan very effective
Effect of pain on lifestyle	Time off work, lack of pleasure in life, but no depression	Has had to take some time off work, mood low
Examination	Slight decrease in light touch over maxillary area	Microvascular decompression scar tender, no sensory abnormalities
MRI	Vessel in contact with the trigeminal nerve on the right but no distortion, no other features	No slippage of Teflon, no new compressions identified

CHAPTER 6

should be called a painful trigeminal neuropathy. Another rare form of facial pain is facial migraine in which the migrainous symptoms are described in the lower part of the face.

Patient 1 has TN with concomitant pain and as she has no neurovascular compression is an idiopathic type. She may have had pre-TN.

Patient 2 describes a classical TN but the recurrent pain no longer has those features. This could be transformed migraine/facial migraine, PIFP, or an early recurrence of TN.

The characteristics of the most common differential diagnoses of TN are shown Table 6.2. Note the differences in key clinical features. Further details are to be found in Chapters 11–15.

6.6 Investigations

MRI is used to determine the aetiology of classical and secondary TN, trigeminal neuropathy, and will on occasion reveal the cause in short-lasting unilateral neuralgiform headache with conjunctival injection and tearing (SUNCT) and other trigeminal autonomic cephalalgia. As a rule, it is negative in PIFP and temporomandibular disorders (note: TN cannot be diagnosed by MRI, because of a common finding of neurovascular compression in asymptomatic people; see Chapters 5 and 7).

Neurophysiological tests, that is, trigeminal reflexes and trigeminal evoked potentials, show abnormalities in secondary TN, painful trigeminal neuropathy, and variably in PIFP. They tend to be negative in classical and idiopathic TN (see Chapter 5).

6.7 Lay summary

TN is defined as a facial pain that comes in severe, short-lived pain attacks on one side of the face and head. These are typically provoked by light touch, wind, eating, speaking, shaving, and similar relatively innocuous mechanical stimuli. Imaging of the trigeminal nerve using MRI may show a blood vessel pressing on the nerve, and is then called classical TN, or it may show a local tumour or changes from multiple sclerosis, and is categorized as secondary TN. If no convincing cause is found, the condition is referred to as idiopathic TN. Many facial pain conditions simulate TN (discussed in Chapters 11–15) but can be distinguished from it by the quality and location of pain, and sometimes by symptoms.

6.8 RECOMMENDED READING

Cruccu G, Finnerup NB, Jensen TS, et al. Trigeminal neuralgia: new classification and diagnostic grading for clinical practice and research. Neurology. 2016;**87**:220–8. doi: 10.1212/WNL.0000000000002840

Table 6.2 Differential diagnosis for trigeminal neuralgia

	Trigeminal neuralgia	SUNA/SUNCT	Painful trigeminal neuropathy	Persistent idiopathic facial pain	Temporomandibular disorder, masticatory
Main pain, frequency, duration, characteristics	Paroxysms <1 sec to 2 min, daily 3–100, remission periods Sharp, stabbing, shooting	Paroxysms <1 sec to 5 min, daily, 3–200, few remissions Sharp, stabbing, shooting	Continuous pain (fluctuating) Burning, throbbing	Continuous but can be intermittent daily for >2 hours Dull, aching, nagging	Continuous but can be some remissions Dull, aching, gnawing
Other pain	Continuous or intermittent pain between paroxysms	None	Occasional spontaneous shooting pains, less severe than continuous pain	Sharp flare-ups, often headache, migraine, other chronic pain	Occasional flare-ups sharp
Location	Anatomical area, mostly unilateral	Anatomical area, mostly unilateral	Anatomical area, mostly unilateral	Poorly localized bilateral not anatomical	Pre-auricular area, ear radiating to temporalis and masseter muscles, can radiate down the neck, can be unilateral
Autonomics	Very rare	Common	None	Rare	None
Provoking factors	Light touch	Cold wind, vibrations, touch	Touch, pressure, cold	Stress	Prolonged chewing

Trigger zones	>90%, small or pinpoint in size	Trigger areas	Occasional, no severe paroxysms triggered from innocuous mechanical stimuli	None	Tender over temporalis and masseter muscles
Cold/ mechanical allodynia	None	None	Common, over large areas within affected dermatomes	Rare	None
Sensory deficits	Rare	Rare	Always, variable in intensity	May be hypoaesthesia	None
Response to CBZ/OXC	>80% initially	Responds better to lamotrigine	Rarely	Some may respond	None
Response to tricyclics/SNRI	Poor	Poor	Good	Partial	Partial

CBZ, carbamazepine; OXC, oxcarbazepine; SNRI, serotonin and norepinephrine reuptake inhibitor; SUNA, short-lasting unilateral neuralgiform headache with autonomic symptoms; SUNCT, short-lasting unilateral neuralgiform headache with conjunctival injection and tearing.

Maarbjerg S, Wolfram F, Heinskou TB, et al. Persistent idiopathic facial pain. Cephalalgia. 2017;**37**:1231–40. doi: 10.1177/0333102416675618

6.9 Continuing professional development

1. What different phenotypes of TN are listed in the current classification?
2. Can a patient have both TN and painful trigeminal neuropathy at the same time?
3. Can you differentiate a temporomandibular disorder and idiopathic TN on the basis of a high-resolution MRI scan?

CHAPTER 7

Classical and idiopathic trigeminal neuralgia

Joanna M. Zakrzewska and Stine Maarbjerg

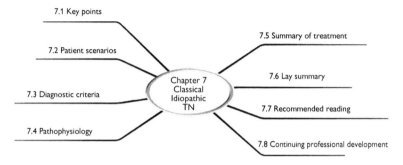

Figure 7.1 Plan of chapter

7.1 KEY POINTS

1. Classical and idiopathic trigeminal neuralgia are termed primary trigeminal neuralgia as no other cause other than compression of the trigeminal nerve is noted in the classical cases. This is noted on magnetic resonance imaging scans.
2. Both these types may report additional dull aching pain which is more constant.
3. The gold standard drugs are carbamazepine and oxcarbazepine.
4. Surgery should be discussed with all patients, half to a third of whom opt for it.
5. Microvascular decompression offers the best and longest period of freedom from pain.
6. Support should be offered in multidisciplinary settings and from patient support groups.

7.2 Patient scenarios

See Table 7.1.

Table 7.1 Two patient scenarios

Features	Patient 1	Patient 2
Sex, age	Male, 50 years	Female, 82 years
Location and radiation	Left maxillary division, intraoral	Right side, starts from forehead radiating down to maxilla but can start from nasolabial area
Characteristics of pain	Paroxysmal, lasting 1–2 sec, episodes can last up to 30 min as a series of stabs with short breaks. Variable number can be every hour	Paroxysms of a few seconds' duration. Several paroxysms as multiple stabs for 20 min with short gaps. Up to 10 a day, refractory period
Severity and quality of pain	Severe (VAS 10/10), shooting, electric shock-like, sharp; 'knife plugged into the mains and then run across the face'; on McGill Pain Questionnaire: fearful, piercing, numbness	Severe (VAS 8/10). Lesser intensity attacks and twinges can occur in same location. Sharp, shooting
Provoking factors	Touching face lightly, talking, eating, brushing teeth, wind	Washing face, cold winds, eating, brushing teeth
Relieving factors	Nil	Nil
Associated features	After the attack may have 30–60 min of uncomfortable numbness, feeling of altered sensation. No autonomic symptoms	No autonomic symptoms
History of pain	Slow onset with pain getting more severe over 2–3 weeks	Memorable onset 4 years ago, episodes of pain with remissions. Currently pain free for 2 months
Effect of pain on life style	Significant, cannot work, depressed, weight loss due to difficulties eating	Lives in fear of pain returning
Clinical examination	Trigger zone in maxillary area, no sensory changes	No active trigger zones, no sensory changes
Investigations	3D MRI: significant compression and distortion of left trigeminal root	3D MRI: no evidence of trigeminal root compression or other changes

3D, three-dimensional; VAS, visual analogue scale.

7.3 Diagnostic criteria

The patients in the two scenarios described in Table 7.1 would both be classified as trigeminal neuralgia (TN), but in patient 1 the magnetic resonance imaging (MRI) scan shows neurovascular compression and so would be called classical TN whereas patient 2 would be termed idiopathic TN. However, both can still be called primary TN. If they have some background pain after the acute attack which lingers on, then these are patients with TN and concomitant pain. The key features are summarized in fig. 7.2. It is crucial to determine the impact on activities of daily living, mood, and sleep as there is evidence that anxiety, depression, and sleep disturbance increase after a diagnosis of TN. It often takes 4–6 years for patients to be seen by specialists and correctly diagnosed.

7.3.1 Classical and idiopathic trigeminal neuralgia

The pain is unilateral in over 90% of patients and located in the distribution of the trigeminal nerve. The right side is slightly more commonly affected as well as the lower part of the face including the mouth. Many patients identify specific trigger

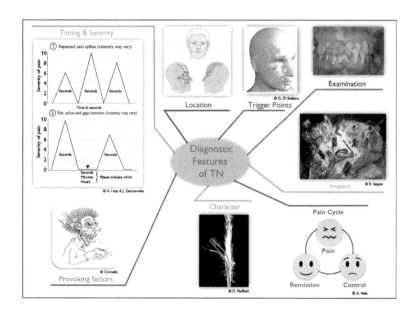

Figure 7.2 Diagnostic criteria for classical TN

Diagram of trigger points shows the principally areas of triggering.

Reproduced from Di Stefano G, Maarbjerg S, Nurmikko T, Truini A, Cruccu G. Triggering trigeminal neuralgia. Cephalalgia. 2018 May;38(6):1049–1056. doi: 10.1177/0333102417721677 with permission from SAGE.

points as shown in fig. 7.2. The first attack of pain is often so severe that patients will remember the circumstances in which it occurred many years later. Most of the attacks are paroxysmal and, on average, patients report 10–50 attacks per day of high-intensity pain. The attacks although single can sometimes become a series of stabs in such rapid succession that they appear to be one long attack. There remains considerable debate around the duration of attacks with some reporting attacks of seconds to 2 minutes, but others reporting much longer attacks. Careful questioning will elicit that there is often a brief refractory period between attacks of pain. Remission periods do occur more frequently at the start of the condition.

It is crucial to listen to the words patients use to describe the pain, often likening it to electric shocks, and shooting or stabbing qualities of pain. Another characteristic feature is that the pain is triggered by light touch such as washing the face, eating, brushing the teeth, or cold wind. Other less common triggers include vibrations and emotional stress. Spontaneous pain is reported in over 60% of patients. Patients may report sensory abnormalities and some of these may be detected on bedside neurological testing. A variety of autonomic features including unilateral conjunctival tearing or injection, runny nose, increased sweating, and miosis/ptosis are reported but they are not noted at each attack.

Although headaches and hypertension are reported, they are not significant comorbidities.

7.3.2 Classical and idiopathic trigeminal neuralgia with concomitant pain

These patients are often younger and more likely to be women than classical TN patients but otherwise the features are the same. This concomitant persistent pain is described as being aching, nagging, and burning in quality and of much lower intensity. It is often present at the start of the condition but may be reported later and can be intermittent. The concomitant pain can last for half a day but in half the patients can be present constantly. More sensory abnormalities are noted in this group.

7.3.3 Imaging and other investigations

High resolution 3-T magnetic resonance imaging (MRI) provides considerable anatomical details and will show whether there is distortion of the nerve by a vessel and/or atrophy of the nerve. Classical TN patients have morphological changes of the trigeminal nerve whereas idiopathic TN patients do not. Despite this, idiopathic TN patients may have a good response to microvascular decompression possibly because a contact between a blood vessel and a nerve may be present. In the future, diffusion tensor imaging may provide more detail of the structural changes and so predict which patients may become pain free after a decompression procedure. Trigeminal afferent damage may be picked up on trigeminal reflex and evoked potential testing, but testing may not be able to distinguish between different types of TN (see Chapter 5).

7.4 Pathophysiology

Changes in myelination especially at the nerve root area have been found on biopsies. The most common theory to date is the ignition hypothesis which results in ephaptic connections. More details are provided in Chapter 3. There may be a different mechanism for the two types of pain and those with concomitant pain have been shown to demonstrate more central sensitization.

7.5 Summary of treatment

7.5.1 Pharmacological therapies

The updated European guidelines on management of primary TN continue to show that carbamazepine and oxcarbazepine remain the gold standard drugs. The main drugs and their average dosages are summarized in fig. 7.3 and more details are to be found in Chapter 9. Drug changes are common due either to lack of efficacy or poor tolerability. Around 40% of patients will use two drugs in order to improve pain control. Some patients will stop drugs during remission periods while others will remain on lowered doses. It is important that patients increase and lower their dosages slowly. Patients will continue to use medications after surgery and attempt to taper off very slowly. There is weak evidence for the addition of botulinum toxin type A injections to standard medications, but there

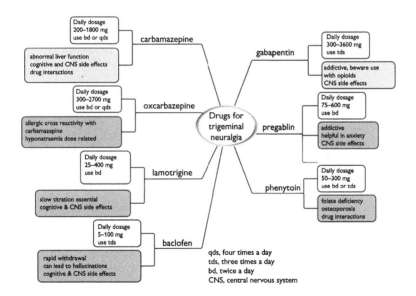

Figure 7.3 Basic drugs used in management of classical TN

is only short follow-up data. For acute flare-ups there is very little evidence but topical lidocaine or an infusion of fosphenytoin may be attempted. Some of the antiseizure medications are available in liquid form. Patients may require admission for rehydration and correction of hyponatraemia due to use of high-dose antiepileptics.

7.5.2 Surgical therapies

The best timing for surgery remains debatable but certainly decreased quality of life and poor tolerability of medication are major determinates.

Patients and their significant others should be involved in the decision process and patients should be informed of the range of surgical treatments early on in their management so they can make more rational choices when not in severe pain. A joint clinic with a neurosurgeon and physician provides an opportunity for patients to be given both points of view and is valued by them. Patient choice varies and from current data the highest number taking up a surgical procedure is around 50% in the UK. Type of surgery performed is not determined by age but by frailty, suitability for general anaesthetic, and other comorbidities. Microvascular decompression of the trigeminal nerve is the most invasive but least destructive procedure and offers the longest period of pain relief, 70% of patients are pain free at 10 years. It is the only procedure associated with a mortality of around 0.3% and with a 0.6% risk of cerebral complications such as stroke, oedema, and haemorrhage. Other available procedures are ablative/destructive. The results and complications based on the European Academy of Neurology guidelines are summarized in fig. 7.4 and in Chapter 10. The numbers of patients used in generating the percentages vary from 51,499 to 289 and the pain-free times have a very wide range but all have at least 3 years of follow-up. Sensory loss can result in corneal hypaesthesia in up to 6.6% or keratitis in up to 1% of patients after ablative procedures.

7.5.3 Other therapies

Fear, anxiety, depression, and isolation can be minimized by providing support from a multidisciplinary team which includes clinical nurse specialists, physiotherapists, and psychologists. Further details are provided in Chapter 16. Contact with support groups can be extremely helpful (see Chapter 17).

7.6 Lay summary

Classical and idiopathic TN are the most common forms of TN and are only distinguished by findings on scans. In scans done in patients with classical TN there are blood vessels distorting or compressing the trigeminal nerve just as it enters the brain within the skull.

Both these types of TN can be associated with some background pain which can be present intermittently or constantly. The gold standard treatment remains carbamazepine and oxcarbazepine, but other medications can be used as shown

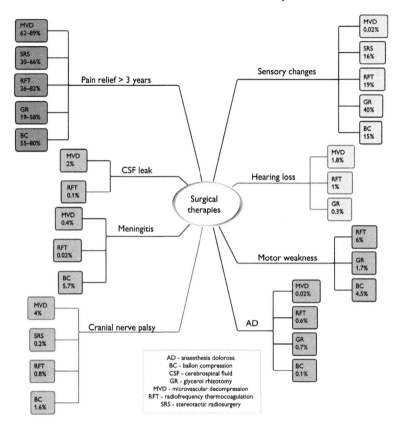

Figure 7.4 Summary of surgical procedures for classical TN

Source data from European Academy of Neurology guideline on trigeminal neuralgia 2019 doi: 0.1111/ene.13950.

in fig. 7.3. The range of surgical options are shown in fig. 7.4. It is important to provide support to improve quality of life.

7.7 RECOMMENDED READING

Haviv Y, Khan J, Zini A, et al. Trigeminal neuralgia (part I): revisiting the clinical phenotype. Cephalalgia. 2015;**36**:730–46. doi: 0333102415611405 [pii];10.1177/0333102415611405

Maarbjerg S, Gozalov A, Olesen J, et al. Trigeminal neuralgia—a prospective systematic study of clinical characteristics in 158 patients. Headache. 2014;**54**:1574–82. doi: 10.1111/head.1244

Zakrzewska JM, Wu J, Mon-Williams M, et al. Evaluating the impact of trigeminal neuralgia. Pain. 2017;**158**:1166–74. doi: 10.1097/j.pain.0000000000000853

7.8 Continuing professional development

1. What is the major difference between classical TN and idiopathic TN?
2. Which of the following statements are true?
   a. Patients can report continuous background pain in classical TN.
   b. Patients with TN have allodynia.
   c. Microvascular decompression is the surgery of choice for idiopathic TN.
   d. The gold standard drug for TN is carbamazepine.
3. When should surgery be offered to patients with TN?

CHAPTER 8

Secondary trigeminal neuralgia

Andrea Truini and Turo Nurmikko

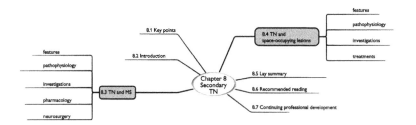

Figure 8.1 Plan of chapter

8.1 KEY POINTS

1. Around 10% of all trigeminal neuralgia (TN) is caused by tumours, arteriovenous malformations (AVMs), or multiple sclerosis.
2. Although patients are often younger and show more sensory deficits compared to those with classical or idiopathic TN, no clinical presentation alone can rule out secondary TN, and magnetic resonance imaging is mandatory.
3. Surgical resection of the tumour or AVM when possible will yield excellent long-term results. Stereotactic radiosurgery is suitable for inoperable tumours but is less effective. Endovascular embolization for AVMs is used mainly as adjunct therapy.
4. Remaining pain can be treated with selective neuroablative palliative procedures and medication.

8.2 Introduction

By definition, any clinically established trigeminal neuralgia (TN) caused by an underlying disease qualifies as secondary TN. International Classification of Headache Disorders, third edition (ICHD-3) and International Classification of Orofacial Pain, first edition (ICOP-1) criteria for the condition are virtually identical. Both underline the usefulness of magnetic resonance imaging (MRI) in detecting the commonest causes (multiple sclerosis (MS), tumour, arteriovenous malformation (AVM)) and recommend trigeminal reflexes and evoked potentials as suitable for patients unable to undergo MRI.

8.3 Trigeminal neuralgia attributed to multiple sclerosis

See Table 8.1 for patient scenario 1.

8.3.1 Clinical features

Diagnostic criteria for secondary trigeminal neuralgia (ICHD-3/ICOP)

A. Recurrent paroxysms of unilateral facial pain fulfilling criteria for TN.

B. Both of the following:
- a. MS has been diagnosed.
- b. An MS plaque at the trigeminal root entry zone or in the pons affecting the intrapontine trigeminal afferents has been demonstrated by MRI, or its presence is suggested by routine electrophysiological studies* showing impairment of trigeminal pathways.

Table 8.1 Patient scenario I

Features	TN attributed to MS
Sex, age	Female, 68 years
Location and radiation	Left V1, V2
Characteristics	Occurs in paroxysms, both spontaneous and evoked. No interparoxysmal pain
Severity and quality of pain	Intense, sharp, visual analogue scale max. 9/10
Provoking factors	Speaking, washing face, eating, coughing, wind
Relieving factors	Nil. Can only tolerate carbamazepine 200 mg/daily with little effect on pain
Associated features	Subjective numbness of face
History of pain	Relapsing–remitting MS diagnosed 12 years ago. First pain attack during a meal at a restaurant 2 months ago
Effect on mental health	Anxious, fearful that new pain is signalling future deterioration of her MS
Effect of pain on lifestyle	Pain more limiting of activities of daily living than problems with gait and balance
Clinical examination	Trigeminal nerve functions: clear reduction in sensitivity to light touch and pinprick in V2. Other: internuclear ophthalmoplegia, dysarthria, unsteady gait, exaggerated lower limb tendon reflexes, plantar extension (all related to MS)

C. Not better accounted for by another ICHD-3/ICOP diagnosis.
(* Neurophysiological recording of trigeminal reflexes and trigeminal evoked potentials.)

Approximately 4% of people with MS report TN in cross-sectional studies but lifetime prevalence appears higher, up to 10%. MS-related TN (MS-TN) affects mainly women (60.5%) with a mean age of onset of 45.4 years. In most patients, it develops years after the diagnosis of MS but in one of six patients, TN is the presenting symptom of MS. Pain is described in terms commonly used for classical and idiopathic TN, and may present as paroxysms only or with additional concomitant continuous or near-continuous interparoxysmal pain (see Chapter 6). In patients with pre-existing MS, the diagnosis is usually straightforward as long as the main differential diagnosis, that of central, non-TN pain, is ruled out. Young patients presenting with new symptoms compatible with TN and showing sensory deficits should raise a suspicion of secondary TN due to MS (Table 8.2), and MRI is essential.

8.3.2 Pathophysiology

The primary mechanism of paroxysmal pain is believed to be focal demyelination of the central terminals of primary afferents traversing the pons on their course to the trigeminal brainstem complex, rendering the nerve fibre susceptible to the same pathogenetic mechanisms deemed to cause classical TN, such as ectopic excitation, high-frequency discharges, and ephaptic transmission. Pontine MS lesions affecting the second-order neurons of the trigeminothalamic tract preferentially lead to non-paroxysmal pain or dysaesthesia, and the condition is then labelled as central pain. It remains an important differential diagnosis for TN associated with MS.

Table 8.2 Comparison of clinical presentation of secondary TN versus classical and idiopathic trigeminal neuralgia

	TN attributed to MS	Classical and idiopathic TN
Age at onset <40 years	>50%*	<5%
Bilateral TN	15–20%	<5%
Sensory deficit on bedside testing	>50%	<20%
History of spontaneous remissions	Uncommon	Common (>60%)

* If associated with sensory change, or is the presenting symptom.

Some patients with MS-TN are found to have prominent neurovascular compression of the trigeminal root on MRI, in addition to an intrapontine demyelinating plaque. The two pathologies may act in concert to generate the pain through a double-crush mechanism, combining inflammatory demyelination with mechanical demyelination of the same first-order neurons. However, the pathogenetic role of neurovascular compression still remains a matter of debate due to conflicting evidence.

8.3.3 Investigations

T2 (or T2 fluid-attenuated inversion recovery (FLAIR))-weighted sequences are required to show areas of focal hyperintensity caused by the demyelinating plaque, commonly found in the dorsal root entry zone, a region rich in myelin (fig. 8.2). Although use of 3.0 T strength is preferable, even 1.5 T MRI will identify them in two-thirds of cases. The routine TN paradigm (see Chapter 5) will also help to depict possible vascular compression/contact and rule out other causes of TN. Trigeminal brainstem reflexes are abnormal in more than 90% of patients with MS-TN (see Chapter 5), which in fact may be useful in the assessment of a MRI-negative patient with TN, especially if younger than 50 years of age.

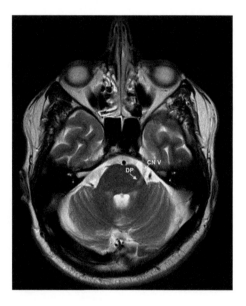

Figure 8.2 Secondary TN due to MS

T2-weighted MRI image showing the trigeminal nerve root (V) and a hyperdense lesion (demyelinating plaque, DP) central to the dorsal root entry zone overlying the intrapontine trigeminal pathway.

8.3.4 Pharmacotherapy

Pharmacological management is in principle the same as for other types of TN (see Chapter 9). There are no adequately powered controlled trials to guide treatment; all data regarding effectiveness and adverse effects come from small comparator trials and observational studies. By common consensus, the sodium channel blockers carbamazepine and oxcarbazepine are recommended as initial treatment for pain paroxysms; lamotrigine is commonly used as second-line treatment or as an add-on. As their effectiveness against concomitant continuous pain is limited, use of pregabalin or gabapentin, or possibly a serotonin and noradrenaline reuptake inhibitor (SNRI) as an add-on can be considered. Baclofen used for MS spasticity could potentially help but no data are available. Topical treatments, especially botulinum toxin, have not been adequately investigated. It should be noted that many MS patients tolerate centrally acting drugs poorly which restricts their optimal use for TN.

8.3.5 Neurosurgery

It is generally agreed that patients who do not respond to medication or cannot attain the therapeutic dosage required should be considered for surgery. Problematically, almost all published data on surgical interventions for MS-TN come from small retrospective case series, leaving unanswered questions about the best neurosurgical approach. Reported outcomes on case series of MS-TN indicate surgical procedures to be less effective long term than in other TN forms. No surgical procedure is able to guarantee a recurrence rate lower than 50% within 3 years. Surgery is therefore limited to providing a medication-free period and repeated surgeries are a frequent event with MS-TN patients. Also, in the subgroup of patients with coexisting demyelination plaque and neurovascular compression, long-term recurrence rates are higher than those observed in classical TN. In general, the effectiveness of microvascular decompression (MVD) in MS-TN does not seem better than what is obtained from neuroablation, which is currently the preferred option. Among neuroablative procedures none has been shown to be superior, with differences seen mainly in frequency of adverse events and onset of therapeutic action (see Chapter 10).

8.4 Trigeminal neuralgia attributed to a space-occupying lesion

Table 8.3 provides the history of a patient with a tumour.

8.4.1 Clinical features

Space-occupying lesions include tumours, AVMs, arteriovenous fistulas, and giant aneurysms. The patient presents with painful paroxysms, both spontaneous and evoked, indistinguishable from classical or idiopathic TN. Concomitant continuous pain may also be present. It is important to make the distinction from painful trigeminal neuropathy (see Chapters 5 and 11). Some patients describe headache or mild motor symptoms. Patients with arteriovenous fistulas may report pulsatile

Table 8.3 Patient scenario 2

Features	TN attributed to a tumour
Sex, age	Female, 68
Location and radiation	Right V2, V3
Characteristics	Occurs in paroxysms, both spontaneous and evoked
Severity and quality of pain	Intense, sharp
Provoking factors	Eating, drinking, speaking, touching face
Relieving factors	Carbamazepine in small doses reduces intensity but not frequency of paroxysms. Cannot tolerate large doses. Added pregabalin affords little benefit
Associated features	Diffuse headache, made worse by lying down
History of pain	First paroxysms 3 months ago, initially infrequently. Currently numerous attacks per day
Effect on mental health	Anxiety, frustration, fear of attacks
Effect of pain on lifestyle	Struggles to eat and drink
Clinical examination	Trigger zones in left nostril, left lower lip. Left corneal reflex weak
MRI	Large cerebellopontine tumour on the right

tinnitus. Sensory deficit is found in 60%, dysaesthesia to touch in 30%, and weakened corneal reflex in 25%. A bruit audible on auscultation over the eyes, temples, or occiput is a hallmark sign of an arteriovenous fistula.

8.4.2 Pathophysiology

In retrospective case series on TN, tumours are reported in 2–12%. They are commonly located in the cerebellopontine angle but when large may extend into the middle cranial fossa, Meckel's cave, or cavernous sinus. Most are non-malignant but metastases or invasively growing nasopharyngeal carcinomas are also encountered (Table 8.4). Pain results from direct compression or displacement of the trigeminal root. The compression may be also indirect, with the tumour pushing an artery or vein against the root. A mass effect from a large supratentorial or posterior fossa tumour has been reported to cause angulation and distortion of the nerve root entry/exit, resulting in TN.

Less than 1% of TN is caused by AVMs found in the posterior fossa (cerebellopontine angle, cerebellar vermis). The mechanisms include direct compression of the root by the feeding artery, nidus, or draining vein (Table 8.4). An enlarged draining vessel of a more remote malformation may also cause the same. An aneurysm localized strategically may lead to increased neural excitability and cause TN.

Other pathologies are rare and somewhat controversial (Table 8.4).

Table 8.4 Aetiology and treatment of space-occupying lesions causing trigeminal neuralgia

	Tumour	AVMs and other vascular abnormalities	Other
Conditions reported as cause of secondary TN	**Posterior fossa** • Vestibular schwannoma (CPA) • Meningioma (CPA) • Meningioma (petroclival) • Epidermoid **Middle fossa** • Trigeminal schwannoma • Pituitary adenoma • Meckel's cave—epidermoid • Meckel's cave—granulomatous diseases • Invasive nasopharyngeal carcinoma • Metastases, lymphoma **Supratentorial with mass effect** • Temporal lobe glioma • Occipital, frontal meningioma **Other** • Osteoid osteoma • Amyloidoma	• AVM • Cavernoma • Venous angioma • Dural and pial arteriovenous fistula	• Basilar invagination • Arnold–Chiari malformation • Genetic (Charcot–Marie–Tooth and others)
Investigations	3D T1W, T2W MRI	3D TOF MRA	
Treatment of cause	• Surgical resection • SRS • Additional MVD if appropriate	• Surgical resection • Endovascular embolization as adjunct • Additional MVD if appropriate	• None
Pain palliation	• Pharmacotherapy • SRS • (BC/TC/GR)	• Pharmacotherapy • SRS	• Pharmacotherapy

3D, three-dimensional; BC, balloon compression; CPA, cerebellopontine angle; GR, glycerol rhizotomy; MVD, microvascular decompression; TC, radiofrequency thermocoagulation; T1W, T1-weighted; T2W, T2-weighted; TOF, time-of-flight; SRS, stereotactic radiosurgery.

8.4.3 Investigations

MRI is uniquely useful in the visualization of tumours (fig. 8.3) and vascular abnormalities and from apparent flow-void signals also the location of AVMs. Digital subtraction angiography or other cerebral angiography is used for detailed characterization of the latter. For the few who cannot have MRI, judicious use of computed tomography, cerebral angiography, and neurophysiological testing (see Chapter 5, fig. 5.14) will in many cases achieve the same.

8.4.4 Treatment

Treatment is primarily surgical. Total resection of a tumour or AVM yields excellent long-term results, comparable to those from MVD. However, after partial resection the approach is highly individualized and may include MVD, stereotactic radiosurgery (SRS), or endovascular embolization. SRS has been shown to reduce the size of epidermal tumours with excellent long-term pain remission. In contrast, one-half of patients with meningiomas and schwannoma experience early pain relief and one-third of them experience a recurrence in the subsequent 2–3 years. SRS is also used exclusively as a pain-relieving technique (see Chapter 10). If medication is needed long term, it follows the same paradigm as in other types of TN (see Chapter 9).

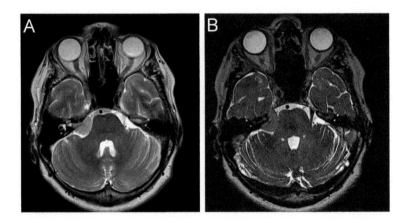

Figure 8.3 Secondary TN due to cerebellopontine angle tumour

(A) T2- and (B) T1-weighted MRI images showing a schwannoma in the cerebellopontine angle encasing the cisternal portion of the trigeminal root on the right.

8.5 Lay summary

TN may be caused by a tumour, AVM (tangle of abnormal blood vessels), or MS. The pain they cause is not different from TN pain in general. Tumours and AVMs compress the trigeminal nerve either directly or indirectly via an enlarged or displaced blood vessel. In MS, small inflammatory patches damage the pain pathways running in the brain and cause them to fire excessively. Modern brain imaging methods readily identify all three conditions. Tumours and AVMs are dealt with surgically, but if pain continues or recurs, medication and Gamma Knife surgery are as effective in controlling it as they are in other forms of TN. MS patients tend not to tolerate TN medication well, and current guidelines recommend early consideration for surgical interventions. MVD has not been shown to be any more effective than less invasive percutaneous needle procedures or stereotactic radiosurgery (SRS) which currently are the preferred options. They can be and also need to be repeated at times to maintain pain relief.

8.6 RECOMMENDED READING

Di Stefano G, Maarbjerg S, Truini A. Trigeminal neuralgia secondary to multiple sclerosis: from the clinical picture to the treatment options. J Headache Pain. 2019;**20**:20. doi: 10.1186/s10194-019-0969-0

Wei Y, Zhao W, Pu C, et al. Clinical features and long-term surgical outcomes in 39 patients with tumor-related trigeminal neuralgia compared with 360 patients with idiopathic trigeminal neuralgia. Br J Neurosurg. 2017;**31**:101–6. doi: 10.1080/02688697.2016.1233321

Yuan Y, Zhang Y, Luo QI, et al. Trigeminal neuralgia caused by brain arteriovenous malformations: a case report and literature review. Exp Ther Med. 2016;**12**:69–80. doi: 10.3892/etm.2016.3277

Zakrzewska JM, Wu J, Brathwaite TS. A systematic review of the management of trigeminal neuralgia in patients with multiple sclerosis. World Neurosurg. 2018;**111**:291–306. doi: 10.1016/j.wneu.2017.12.147

8.7 Continuing professional development

1. A patient with known MS and TN refractory to pharmacotherapy has MRI which shows distinct compression of the trigeminal root, ipsilateral to the pain. What surgical treatment or treatments would you recommend?
2. Following partial resection and endovascular embolization of an AVM, the patient complains of less intense but frequent TN paroxysms. What treatment options do you have?

CHAPTER 9

Treatment of trigeminal neuralgia: Pharmacological

Giulia Di Stefano, Turo Nurmikko, and Joanna M. Zakrzewska

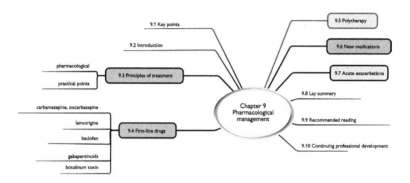

Figure 9.1 Plan of chapter

9.1 KEY POINTS

1. Optimal pharmacological management of trigeminal neuralgia requires teamwork, involving a physician and a pain nurse, with rapid access to a neurosurgeon. In specialized settings, multidisciplinary teams may be involved.
2. First-line pharmacological options are carbamazepine and oxcarbazepine.
3. Second-line medications include lamotrigine, gabapentin, pregabalin, baclofen, and botulinum toxin A.
4. Drug combinations can be beneficial, especially in patients with concomitant continuous pain, but polypharmacy should be avoided and surgical options considered instead.
5. Severe exacerbations may require in-hospital infusions of fosphenytoin alongside rehydration and other measures.

9.2 Introduction

The general recommendation is to commence the treatment of trigeminal neuralgia (TN) with medication and consider surgical procedures in patients who are refractory to pharmacotherapy. Nevertheless, the possibilities of surgical management should be discussed with the patient early on to allow them an informed opinion of when and why to consider the option. The point of transition from pharmacotherapy to surgical therapy will inevitably vary greatly from patient to patient. There are no strong clinical arguments to follow because studies comparing medical and surgical options directly are still lacking, and no clinical or neuroimaging features have been shown to dictate the timing of first surgery. Of note, trade-off studies indicate that some patients would have opted for early surgery and equally, global neurosurgical practice is moving in the same direction. It remains the responsibility of the managing doctor to ensure the patient is aware of both pharmacological and neurosurgical options, thus allowing an informed decision about the choice of treatment.

9.2.1 Before treatment

Prior to commencement of pharmacological treatment, there are several points to take into account (Table 9.1). In general, this includes providing the patient with information regarding the rationale of pharmacotherapy, expected treatment outcome (including the need to adjust medication for optimal outcome), adverse effects, who to contact if needed, and advice on drug interactions or planned pregnancy. It is important to identify any such drug interactions that necessitate avoidance of a drug, or careful observation if one is prescribed. It is useful to do a laboratory work-up and in some patients an electrocardiogram (ECG) may be needed. Multidisciplinary assessment has many benefits but is not always possible; at a minimum, a close collaboration between the physician responsible for the patient's pharmacological management and the neurosurgeon is needed.

It is helpful for the clinician to signal to the patient that the distress caused by TN is well established and that this can be improved by a multidisciplinary approach using a caring approach and building up trust with the patient. This will involve non-pharmacological support (see Chapter 16) and support groups (see Chapter 17), including further evidence-based information.

It should be underlined that side effects may significantly weaken patient compliance even when pain control is entirely satisfactory. It is worth remembering that all antiepileptic drugs increase the risk of suicidal ideation and behaviour.

9.3 Principles of treatment

9.3.1 Pharmacological considerations

While carbamazepine or oxcarbazepine are first-line medications for TN, they are best avoided in certain conditions and prescribed with extra care in others

Table 9.1 Pre-prescription considerations

Medication	Phenotype suitability	Avoid	Caution	Baseline tests	Advice to patient	Note
First line						
Carbamazepine (CBZ)	Best for TN-PP; effect less certain for TN-CCP	Hypersensitivity reaction to OXC or LTG, AV conduction disorders (unless paced), history of bone marrow depression, acute porphyria	History of hypersensitivity reaction to any drug, major cardiac disease, major hepatic/renal disease, glaucoma; old age	Full blood count, liver and renal function tests Asian ancestry: consider testing for HLA-B*1502 allele ECG	Report rash, fever, other hypersensitivity signs immediately Initial sedative side effects likely, will disappear Risk of suicidal ideation/ behaviour Discontinuation: avoid abrupt withdrawal Seek advice if on contraceptive pill or plan pregnancy	Poor balance, caution. Indoors—vitamin D; ensure dietary calcium intake. Folate deficiency long-term use Ensure arrangement for nurse support/ follow-up Promote use of pain diaries
Oxcarbazepine (OXC)	As above	Hypersensitivity reaction to OXC or LTG, AV conduction disorders (unless paced)	History of hypersensitivity reactions to any drug, major cardiac disease, severe hepatic impairment, reduced renal function (creatine clearance <30 mL/min)	As above	As above	As above

(continued)

Table 9.1 Continued

Medication	Phenotype suitability	Avoid	Caution	Baseline tests	Advice to patient	Note
Second line						
Lamotrigine (LTG)	Best suited for add-on treatment, both TN-PP and TN-CCP	Hypersensitivity reaction to OXC or LTG	History of hypersensitivity reactions to any drug, Parkinson's disease, severe hepatic/renal impairment	Full blood count, liver and renal function tests Asian ancestry: consider testing for HLA-B*1502 allele	Report rash, fever, other hypersensitivity signs immediately Risk of suicidal ideation/ behaviour Avoid abrupt withdrawal Seek advice if pregnancy planned	Arrangement for nurse support/follow-up Promote use of pain diaries
Gabapentin (GBP)	Uncertain efficacy in TN-PP; best suited for add-on in TN-CCP		Diabetes mellitus; history of psychotic illness or substance misuse; risk of respiratory depression in those with compromised respiratory function, respiratory or neurological disease, renal impairment, and elderly	Renal function tests	Initial sedative side effects likely, will disappear Risk of suicidal ideation/ behaviour Avoid abrupt withdrawal	As above

Pregabalin	As above		Congestive heart disease, encephalopathy (or risk of one), renal impairment	Renal function tests	As above	As above
Baclofen (BACL)	All types of TN (limited data available)	Conditions associated with muscle hypotonia	Cerebrovascular disease; diabetes; elderly; epilepsy; history of peptic ulcer; hypertonic bladder sphincter; Parkinson's disease; psychiatric illness; respiratory impairment; renal impairment; hepatic impairment		Risk of epileptic seizures, sedative	As above
Botulinum toxin A	All types of TN (limited data available)		Neuromuscular disease, history of dysphagia or aspiration, elderly Risk of angle closure glaucoma injections in first and second divisions		Look out for any signs of spread of toxin. May induce local muscle weakness (facial asymmetry)	May need to inject bilaterally to avoid asymmetry

AV, atrioventricular; TN-CCP, trigeminal neuralgia with concomitant continuous pain (TN2); TN-PP, trigeminal neuralgia, purely paroxysmal (TN1).

(Table 9.1). The phenotype of TN likely plays a role although the data are limited. Patients with continuous concomitant pain between paroxysms may not respond to carbamazepine or oxcarbazepine (or another sodium channel blocker) alone and co-medication with an agent better suited for non-paroxysmal neuropathic pain may be added on early (e.g. a gabapentinoid, tricyclic antidepressant, or serotonin and norepinephrine reuptake inhibitor).

Carbamazepine and oxcarbazepine are contraindicated in patients with atrioventricular block. Other specific contraindications to the use of sodium channel blockers include severe arrhythmias and allergic reactions.

Hypersensitivity reactions that are seen with carbamazepine, oxcarbazepine, and lamotrigine range from maculopapular exanthema with mild associated systemic symptoms to life-threatening toxic reactions, Stevens–Johnson syndrome/toxic epidermal necrolysis(SJS/TEN) and drug reaction with eosinophilia and systemic symptoms (DRESS). The mortality associated with these conditions is estimated at 5–30%. These are associated with the human leucocyte antigen (HLA)-B*1502 genotype especially in Chinese, Malaysian, and Thai populations; indeed, the US Food and Drug Administration recommends pre-emptive HLA genotyping for patients with Asian ancestry who are at highest risk for the development of SJS. Some European countries have adopted similar recommendations. Carbamazepine-induced hypersensitivity reactions have been associated with other HLA variants (HLA-B*1511, HLA-A*3101). The usefulness of the test is compromised by its suboptimal sensitivity and specificity.

There is a high degree of cross-reactivity (40–80%) between the carbamazepine and oxcarbazepine (and up to 50% with lamotrigine).

Drug–drug interactions

Carbamazepine is a strong cytochrome P450 (CYP)-3A4 inducer and can reduce the effectiveness of oral contraceptives and interfere with the action of warfarin and potentially direct oral anticoagulants. Oxcarbazepine is a weak CYP3A4 inducer but it may interact in a similar way in high doses (1200 mg/day). In countries where oxcarbazepine is licensed for TN, it may be a safer option to start with. The main elimination of lamotrigine is via metabolism by uridine glucuronosyltransferase (UGT) which is weakly induced by carbamazepine and oxcarbazepine. The metabolism of several antidepressants involves CYP3A4 and the UGT system, therefore a potential clinically meaningful interaction may happen. However, relevant literature is limited and it is not clear how clinically important these interactions are. They should be kept in mind if the therapeutic response is found to be suboptimal, or side effects become a problem. Pregabalin and gabapentin, eliminated via a renal route, are devoid of interactions that could affect TN therapy (although are not usually suitable as the only medication, see section 9.4.4). When prescribing for patients with polypharmacy, it is advisable to check potential interactions from reliable sources, such as national drug formularies.

Women of fertile age should be reminded that carbamazepine and oxcarbazepine as hepatic enzyme-inducing agents interfere with the metabolism of combined hormonal contraceptives and incur a risk of failed contraception. Lamotrigine does not reduce the effectiveness of hormonal contraception but uniquely an ethinyloestradiol/levonorgestrel combination reduces the concentration of circulating lamotrigine, while progesterone increases it.

Recent literature suggests that there is a low risk of major congenital malformations from carbamazepine, oxcarbazepine, and lamotrigine taken during pregnancy with the latter being the lowest risk. But there are risks for other adverse outcomes (e.g. spontaneous miscarriage, haemorrhage) although most of the studies are done in patients taking antiepileptics for seizures, not for other reasons. The data regarding pregabalin and gabapentin are limited and conflicting.

Pharmacological treatment of TN secondary to multiple sclerosis is challenging, owing to the patients' poor tolerability of centrally acting drugs. While also in this patient group carbamazepine and oxcarbazepine are considered first-line drugs, they may induce intolerable side effects and necessitate consideration for an early neurosurgical intervention. Other recommended drugs (Table 9.1) tend to be similarly sedative. European experts' consensus suggests that baclofen may be useful in patients with multiple sclerosis. Such patients are often already taking baclofen to reduce spasticity and may achieve control of symptoms with little or no added carbamazepine.

9.3.2 Practical points

It is important to stress to the patient that the drugs are preventive and are to be taken regularly. Compliance is improved if the patient is told that their medication will initially induce sedative side effects, but these tend to significantly reduce in the following weeks. All oral medications suitable for TN should be started at low doses and built up stepwise to the level that controls pain, or when troublesome side effects appear (see Table 9.3 later in this chapter). Some are available as liquid preparations which can be used if swallowing is difficult. The older the patient, the more conservative one should be with the prescribed doses. It has been suggested that women in general are less tolerant of high doses than men. As in TN, especially in early stages, remissions occur, and patients should be encouraged to adapt the dosages accordingly. Lowering the dose is advised over several days after they have been pain free for a month. If side effects have necessitated dose reduction which then leads to pain recurrence, cautious dose incrementation may be tried as adaptation to side effects tends to occur. Patients should be advised not to stop medication abruptly. In case of a drug-induced hypersensitivity syndrome, the withdrawal by necessity will have to happen rapidly but always under clinical observation. Long-term use of antiepileptics can result in osteoporosis so calcium levels need to be checked. Bone densitometry may be required, especially in older women who are at risk of falls.

Table 9.3 Commonly used drugs for trigeminal neuralgia

Drug	Mechanism of action	Starting dose	Usual dose range	Titration	Main adverse events
Carbamazepine	Voltage-gated sodium channel blocker	200–400 mg	200–1200 mg	Increase by 200 mg every third day	Drowsiness, ataxia, dizziness, skin reactions, nausea, vomiting, blood dyscrasia, cognitive impairment
Oxcarbazepine	Voltage-gated sodium channel blocker	300 mg	300–1800 mg	300 mg every 3 days	Drowsiness, ataxia, dizziness, hyponatraemia, cognitive impairment
Lamotrigine	Acting at voltage-sensitive sodium channels, stabilizes neural membranes and inhibits the release of excitatory neurotransmitters	25 mg	25–400 mg	25 mg every 2 weeks but can increase weekly after first 4 weeks	Dizziness, nausea, blurred vision, ataxia, cognitive impairment, skin reactions
Baclofen	GABA-B receptor agonist, depresses excitatory neurotransmission	10 mg	40–60 mg	5 mg every third day	Drowsiness, dizziness, gastrointestinal discomfort, loss of muscle tone, severe withdrawal symptoms if stopped too quickly
Gabapentin	Binding to alpha2-delta subunits of voltage-gated calcium channel	300 mg	300–3000 mg	300 mg every third day	Drowsiness, unsteadiness, weight gain, peripheral oedema, cognitive impairment
Pregabalin	Binding to alpha2-delta subunits of voltage-gated calcium channel	75 mg	150–600 mg	75 mg every 3 days	Drowsiness, unsteadiness, weight gain, peripheral oedema, cognitive impairment
Botulinum neurotoxin type A (ona-, abo-, incobotulinum toxin)	TRPV1 receptor block reducing local release of antinociceptive neuropeptides such as substance P, and calcitonin gene-related peptide	Depends on preparation	Depends on preparation	NA	Transient facial weakness, focal oedema

PAIN DIARY

Patient's name: Hospital Number:

Date of visit:

At the end of each day please record your pain severity and ability to do activities according to the definitions
a) How intense (severe) is the pain?
        On a scale of 0–10, where 0 = no pain, 10 = worse pain ever
b) How much has the pain interfered with your daily activities?
        On a scale of 0–10, where 0 = no pain, 10 = worse pain ever
c) How severe are the side effects of the drugs? You may wish to specify what they are
        On a scale of 0 = 10, where 0 = no side effecs, 10 = severe side effects that stop all activities
d) Please enter number of tablets per day and which ones, by initial.

Carbamazepine (Tegretol)	100mg (C1)	Lamotrogine (Lamactil)	25/25/100 mg (L)
Carbamazepine (Tegretol)	200mg (C2)	Gabapentin (Neurontin)	300mg/600mg (G)
Carbamazepine retard	200/400mg (CR)	Nortriptyline (Allegron)	10/20/30/40mg (N)
Oxcarbazepine (Trileptal)	300mg (OXC)	Fluoxetine (Prozac)	20mg (P)
Baclofen (Lioresal)	10 mg (B)	Pregablin (Lyrica)	25/50/75/100/150/300mg (PG)

PROPOSED DOSAGE SCHEDULES
The times are just a guideline.

Days/weeks	7.00 a.m.	12 MD	5.00 p.m.	11.00 p.m.
21.7.2020	C2: 200mg	C2: 200mg		C2: 200mg
	G 600mg	G 600mg		G 600mg
24.7.2020	C2: 200mg			C2: 200mg
	G 600mg	G 600mg		G 600mg

Date	Pain	Activity	No. Tabs	Side Effects	Date	Pain	Activity	No. Tabs	Side Effects

Figure 9.2 Example of a pain diary

Use of pain diaries is recommended as a means of quantification of the severity of the condition which will help the clinician to estimate the effective target dosage (fig. 9.2 is an example of a pain diary). Both frequency and severity of paroxysms should be recorded—this is particularly important when the medication is started. The severity of each paroxysm is rated by the patient on an 11-point numerical rating scale ranging from 0 to 10 (0 is no pain and 10 is the maximum pain imaginable), with all scores averaged over 24 hours. Recording of adverse effects over the same time period would allow more clinical discretion with regard to dose escalation. Patients could also record their ability to carry out activities.

Nurse specialists trained in the management of TN can offer a very useful complementary clinical service that improves patient experience by providing advice and ensuring smooth implementation of treatment plans. Their role is important in maintaining patient adherence to treatment and facilitating rapid action when necessary. There is emerging evidence that this activity is highly cost-effective.

9.4 First-line pharmacological treatment

See Table 9.2 for patient scenario 1.

9.4.1 Carbamazepine and oxcarbazepine

Carbamazepine (200–1200 mg/day) and oxcarbazepine (600–1800) are the first-choice medical treatments for pain control in patients with TN (Table 9.3).

Although not supported by high-level randomized controlled trials, their efficacy is exemplary, with a meaningful pain control in almost 90% of patients, to the point that early refractoriness to these drugs should prompt steps to reaffirm the diagnosis. Their efficacy is related to extensive blockade of voltage-gated sodium

Table 9.2 Patient scenario 1	
Features	Choice of medication
Sex, age	Female, 68 years
Location and radiation	Left V1–3 and intraoral
Characteristics of pain	Paroxysmal, up to 30 attacks per day each lasting a few seconds
Severity and quality of pain	Severe (visual analogue scale 8–10); sharp, shooting
Provoking factors	Brushing teeth, eating, touching face
Relieving factors	Carbamazepine
History of pain	Sharp and shooting pain first started 3 years ago and the diagnosis TN made. Attacked controlled with carbamazepine but only with doses causing sedative side effects. Few weeks ago, had a fall and was seen in emergency unit, no fractures, found to have a sodium level of 132 mmol/L. Has had falls in the past prior to TN
Other relevant history	On regular alendronic acid, Adcal-D3® for osteoporosis
Effect of pain on lifestyle	Significant impact on activities of daily living, mild depression
Clinical examination	Neurological examination was normal
Investigations/management	Magnetic resonance imaging, with specifications optimized for identification of the TN aetiology, shows contact more than compression without any morphological changes on the trigeminal root. The second-line drug lamotrigine was tried with a slow titration. The possibility of gamma knife or percutaneous ganglion lesion was discussed

channels in a frequency-dependent manner, which results in the stabilization of hyperexcited neuronal membranes and inhibition of repetitive firing. In the clinical setting, most treatment failures are not due to lack of drug effectiveness, but undesired side effects that necessitate either discontinuation of the drug or reduction of dosage to a suboptimal level.

The effective dose in patients with TN may be less than that required to treat patients with epilepsy. Carbamazepine in some patients may be effective with a dosage of 100 mg two to three times a day. For the remaining patients, the daily dose should be increased by 200 mg every third day until adequate pain relief is established or until intolerable side effects prevent further upward titration. Typical maintenance doses range from 300 to 800 mg/day divided into two to four daily doses; doses up to 1800 mg may be required. Slow-release preparations are available but there are no studies to compare them with the conventional forms.

Oxcarbazepine is an acceptable alternative to carbamazepine and is initiated at 150 mg twice daily and increased as tolerated by 300 mg every 3 days until pain relief is accomplished. Maintenance doses range between 300 and 600 mg twice daily or four times daily. Maximum doses are up to 2700 mg. If there is no efficacy from carbamazepine, treatment can be switched directly to the equipotent dose of oxcarbazepine (carbamazepine 200 mg equals oxcarbazepine 300 mg).

The well-established effectiveness of first-line drugs is compromised by low tolerability. The most common side effects are dizziness, diplopia, ataxia, and elevation of transaminases that cause withdrawal from treatment in a significant percentage of patients (about 20%). When tested, cognitive performance is affected in a high percentage of people on either drug.

Both carbamazepine and oxcarbazepine may cause clinically significant hyponatraemia which is dose related. Sodium levels should be monitored during the treatment, especially in patients using high doses. Diuretics may add to the risk of hyponatraemia. Reduction of the dose or discontinuation of the offending drug and introduction of second-line alternatives may suffice; surgical options should also be considered. When this is not possible, sodium chloride capsules in persistent cases of hyponatraemia are advocated by some authors but fluids should not be restricted.

Especially in the first weeks of therapy, mild leucopenia occurs commonly but requires no action. Severe blood dyscrasia (agranulocytosis, thrombocytopenia, or aplastic anaemia occurs in a small minority, estimated at 0.06%); there is no evidence to suggest that routine monitoring is worthwhile. Liver enzyme elevation happens in a majority but has little clinical relevance, and severe hepatopathy is rare in people with no coexisting liver disease. Non-experts need to be aware of this. There have been reports of lymphadenopathy and systemic lupus erythematosus relating to carbamazepine. Severe hypersensitivity reactions are known to happen.

It is advisable to determine the full blood count, electrolytes, liver function tests (once), and ECG after the first few weeks of treatment. The latter is advisable as atrioventricular conduction abnormalities may develop during early stages of treatment.

When first-line drugs become ineffective or result in poor tolerability, lamotrigine, baclofen, gabapentin, pregabalin, and botulinum toxin type A may be considered either alone or as add-on therapy. It should be emphasized that the quality of evidence for their use is low or very low.

9.4.2 Lamotrigine

Lamotrigine acts at voltage-sensitive sodium channels, stabilizes neural membranes, and inhibits the release of excitatory neurotransmitters. It is important to start with very low doses and escalate slowly. This limits its use in acute flare-ups. A skin rash (7–10% of cases) can occur but does not necessarily indicate an allergy. With severe rash, desquamation or SJS/TEN, or DRESS, prompt discontinuation is required (see section 9.3.2). The slower the titration, the less likely it is that these side effects will occur.

9.4.3 Baclofen

Baclofen is a gamma-aminobutyric acid type B (GABA-B) receptor agonist and thus depresses excitatory neurotransmission. Baclofen is initiated at 10 mg daily and may be gradually increased by 5 mg every third day. Caution is needed when baclofen is combined with other central nervous system depressants. Tricyclic antidepressants may potentiate the effect of baclofen. Potential side effects include drowsiness, dizziness, gastrointestinal discomfort, and loss of muscle tone. It is often used in patients with multiple sclerosis who take it for spasticity. Abrupt discontinuation may cause seizures and hallucinations.

9.4.4 Gabapentin and pregabalin

Gabapentin and pregabalin are alpha2-delta ligands that inhibit the activity of the voltage-gated calcium channel at the presynaptic level, thus reducing the synaptic release of neurotransmitters and the activation of the postsynaptic neuron. Gabapentin is initiated at 300 mg daily and may be gradually increased by 300 mg every 3 days as tolerated with doses as high as 3700mg being used. Pregabalin is initiated at 75 mg daily and may be gradually increased up to a final dose of 300 mg per day divided between two doses. These antiepileptic drugs may produce relatively minor side effects including dizziness, somnolence, and confusion. Weight gain and leg oedema are common. Allergic reactions are rare but it should be noted that there is cross-reactivity between pregabalin and gabapentin.

9.4.5 Botulinum neurotoxin type A

Botulinum neurotoxin type A injected into the skin of the painful area inhibits release of neuropeptides involved in central and peripheral sensitization, such as substance P, glutamate, and calcitonin gene-related peptide, and blocks TRPV1 channels. A further potential mechanism is inhibition of trigeminal ganglion cell sodium channel activity, following transportation of the toxin from the injection site. It is reported that after botulinum toxin injections the pain relief lasts several months but all the randomized controlled trials are of short duration and many patients remain on systemic medications. Generally considered safe, the main side effect is a transient weakness of the facial muscles in the injected area. Note that there are several formulations on the market with different properties, and with different dose recommendations.

9.5 Polytherapy

As shown in Table 9.4, patient scenario 2, medications have been added on without due consideration of the optimal dosage levels, tolerability, and potential interaction. Many patients will use multiple medications before deciding on the one that provides maximum efficacy and best tolerability. If using polytherapy each drug should first be used to its maximum potential and addition of a second drug should result in a review of the first medication. It may be possible to use lower dosages of both drugs. In the long term, a quarter of patients may use

Table 9.4 Patient scenario 2

Features	Multiple drug use
Sex, age	Male, 68 years
Location and radiation	Third division unilateral
Characteristics of pain	Paroxysmal pain, up to 20 attacks per day. Classical TN diagnosed 4 years earlier. Remissions periods of a few weeks only
Severity and quality of pain	Severe (visual analogue scale on average 7/10)
Current problem	Increasing pain, side effects of medication
Current treatment	4 years carbamazepine retard 300 mg at night 4 years gabapentin 900 mg three times a day 3 years phenytoin 300 mg at night Oxcarbazepine 600 mg twice a day, 300 mg later afternoon 6 months baclofen 40 mg daily in divided doses Significant side effects, unsteadiness, dizziness, tiredness, decreased concentration, double vision Difficult to determine which drug may be effective
Effect of pain on lifestyle	Anxiety and depression, significant interference with quality of life and activities of daily living, fear of severe attacks
Clinical examination	Left side poor oral hygiene with build-up of calculus round teeth in lower left quadrant

polytherapy. After a couple of treatment failures, the best course of action is to consider surgical intervention.

9.6 New medications

Among the voltage-gated sodium channels blockers, eslicarbazepine acetate, a third-generation antiepileptic drug belonging to the dibenzazepine group, has so far been tested in patients with TN in an open-label study only. Studies on epilepsy suggest it could be better tolerated than either carbamazepine or oxcarbazepine but its efficacy in TN remains uncertain until randomized controlled trials have been conducted.

Vixotrigine, a new Nav1.7 selective sodium channel blocker, is under development and, thanks to its selectivity, might produce significant pain relief without inducing side effects related to central nervous system depression. Nav1.7 has been validated as a key pain target by human genetic linkage, as gain-of-function mutations are linked to a severe chronic pain syndrome, whereas loss-of-function mutations lead to the inability to feel pain. A phase II randomized controlled trial with vixotrigine showed promising, preliminary findings on the average daily pain score and a favourable adverse events profile, although it was negative for the primary endpoint. Further phase III studies are needed.

The development of new selective sodium channel blockers has been encouraged by the recent discovery of an association between neuropathic pain and rare variants in genes encoding voltage-gated sodium channels. In patients with familial TN, rare variants of genes encoding different voltage-gated channels and TRP channels have been identified.

9.7 Acute exacerbations

Patients with TN may suffer from acute exacerbations (flare-ups) characterized by a very high attack frequency and severity, often leading to dehydration and anorexia because intake of fluids and food can trigger paroxysmal pain. In addition, oral hygiene might be poor because brushing teeth triggers pain. See patient scenario 3 in Table 9.5.

During acute exacerbations, in-hospital treatment is sometimes required for rehydration and drug titration. Pain relief can provide a window for adjustment of oral preventive medication and can be of help until neurosurgical intervention is arranged. Opioids are not effective in safe doses and should be avoided. In severe cases, intravenous infusion of fosphenytoin or lidocaine under cardiac monitoring is used in many centres although evidence comes from case series only. It has been suggested that a single dose of subcutaneous sumatriptan 3 mg can be used similarly, but the data are limited. Injection of lidocaine with or without adrenaline followed by bupivacaine into identified trigger points can provide a few hours of pain relief. It can be repeated daily until the oral medications take effect. Topical

Table 9.5 Patient scenario 3

Features	Acute TN
Sex, age	Male, 59 years
Pain history	Classical TN 10-year history, remission periods of 1–2 years Current recurrence in March of severe pain worse to date
Medications	In the past used pregabalin and gabapentin which were not helpful Carbamazepine up to 1600 mg has always been helpful
Current crisis	In March added lamotrigine June very severe pain, unable to eat, on carbamazepine 1600 mg, lamotrigine 400 mg
Magnetic resonance imaging	No lesions and no neurovascular compression
Management	Treatment of acute exacerbation with intravenous infusion of fosphenytoin after hospital admission and under cardiac monitoring

lidocaine ointments or sprays can reduce triggering of attacks. The evidence is anecdotal.

A summary of treatments is shown in fig. 9.3.

9.8 Lay summary

Before drug therapy for TN is initiated, the patient should be informed of the rationale of pharmacotherapy, expected treatment outcome (including the need to adjust medication for optimal outcome), adverse effects, who to contact if needed, and, when relevant, possible drug interactions or impact on planned pregnancy. Serious allergic reactions are rare but possible and therefore each patient must be educated about the symptoms and signs that may herald one. Severe heart diseases, and liver or kidney disorders, may necessitate reduced doses or abstaining from prescribing altogether. Clinical and psychological support should be available from a dedicated pain nurse and quick access to a neurosurgeon must be ensured. Blood tests and an ECG are needed at the start of treatment, depending on the chosen drug. First-line options are carbamazepine or oxcarbazepine; if needed, other drugs such as lamotrigine, gabapentin, pregabalin, or baclofen may be combined with them. Occasionally, they may be used as sole medication, if the first-line drugs fail and have to be discontinued. Almost all drugs cause early sedation and have a cognitive impact which disappears or attenuates in a matter of weeks. Recently, botulinum toxin A injections into the painful face area have shown effectiveness. Despite many pharmacological options, drug

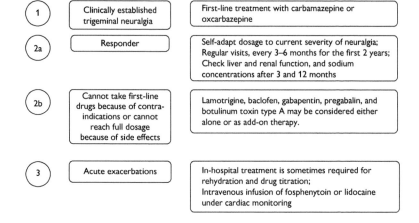

Figure 9.3 Algorithm of main treatments

treatment ultimately fails in a substantial percentage of patients, and surgical solutions should be explored.

9.9 RECOMMENDED READING

Di Stefano G, Yuan JH, Cruccu G, et al. Familial trigeminal neuralgia – a systematic clinical study with a genomic screen of the neuronal electrogenisome. Cephalalgia. 2020;**40**:767–77. doi: 10.1177/0333102419897623

Moore D, Chong MS, Shetty A, et al. A systematic review of rescue analgesic strategies in acute exacerbations of primary trigeminal neuralgia. Br J Anaesth. 2019;**123**:e385–96. doi: 10.1016/j.bja.2019.05.026

Zakrzewska JM, Palmer J, Morisset V, et al. Safety and efficacy of a Nav1.7 selective sodium channel blocker in patients with trigeminal neuralgia: a double-blind, placebo-controlled, randomised withdrawal phase 2a trial. Lancet Neurol. 2017;**16**:291–300. doi: 10.1016/S1474-4422(17)30005-4

9.10 Continuing professional development

1. What are the first-line drugs for TN?
2. What are the main side effects of the antiepileptics and why do they occur?
3. How would you manage an acute flare-up of TN and what would be your indication for admission?
4. Would you maintain a patient on the same dose and drug in the long term?

CHAPTER 10

Treatment of trigeminal neuralgia: Surgical

Introduction
Joanna M. Zakrzewska

Microvascular decompression
Kim J. Burchiel, Raymond F. Sekula Jr, and Marc Sindou

Stereotactic radiosurgery
Jean Régis and Constantin Tuleasca

Percutaneous/ablative procedures
Imran Noorani and Owen Sparrow

Other posterior fossa procedures
Kim J. Burchiel

Other procedures
Joanna M. Zakrzewska

Decision-making
Joanna M. Zakrzewska

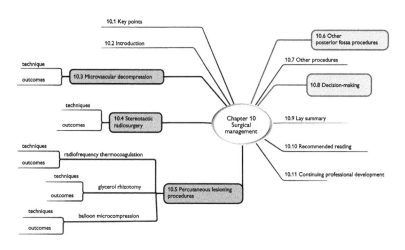

Figure 10.1 Plan of chapter

10.1 KEY POINTS

1. Surgery for trigeminal neuralgia is reserved for patients refractory to medical treatment.
2. Microvascular decompression is the most definitive surgical option for suitable patients providing the highest long-term pain relief period.
3. Microvascular decompression has a small risk of mortality and minor immediate short-term complications but few permanent complications with a very low risk of sensory changes.
4. Stereotactic radiosurgery is the least invasive procedure with similar pain relief periods to other percutaneous procedures but may not be suitable for many patients as repeat procedures (i.e. greater than two) result in significant morbidity.
5. Percutaneous procedures include glycerol rhizolysis, radiofrequency thermocoagulation, and balloon compression performed at the Gasserian ganglion or retrogasserian level.
6. Percutaneous procedures are particularly suited to older and/or less medically fit patients and can be repeated. They provide a few years of pain relief with varying degrees of sensory loss.
7. Internal neurolysis and partial sensory rhizotomy are open ablative techniques used in patients without neurovascular conflict which result in sensory loss.
8. All patients should be informed of the range of surgical procedures as shared decision-making will improve patient satisfaction.

10.2 Introduction

This chapter will cover the range of surgical procedures that are potentially available (fig. 10.1). Although systematic reviews concerning these procedures have been performed, there are still no high-quality randomized controlled trials of any of the procedures or a comparison between different ones. Most of the data is retrospective, very few prospective studies have been reported with independent observers and using validated outcome measures. Although the primary outcome measure is pain relief, some complications such as sensory loss can result in a significant impact on quality of life which will require further management (see Chapters 11 and 16). The data in this chapter represent the best available data albeit low in terms of evidence. At the end of the chapter, a section on decision-making which includes several patient scenarios is included. You will be able to reflect on which procedures would be possible for each patient. Not all patients with trigeminal neuralgia (TN) will require surgery.

10.3 Microvascular decompression

10.3.1 Introduction

Although a variety of surgical procedures are effective in the relief of TN pain, microvascular decompression (MVD) remains an excellent choice for some patients due to its superior durability and avoidance of sensory deficits when performed without complications and intentional trauma to the nerve.

Clearly, the indications for MVD should be based on an affirmative diagnosis of TN, and the demonstration of pathologic neurovascular compression (NVC) on magnetic resonance imaging (MRI). Although MVD is generally considered the 'gold standard' for the surgical treatment of TN, all patients with TN are not candidates for MVD surgery, particularly as there are (valuable) surgical alternative methods such as percutaneous lesioning techniques or stereotactic radiosurgery (SRS).

As discussed in Chapters 11–15, there are a multitude of causes of facial pain. The tendency to make an 'imaging diagnosis' of TN based on an MRI finding of NVC may sometimes lead clinicians and patients down the wrong diagnostic and therapeutic pathway. Many patients with facial pain are found to have incidental vascular compression of the trigeminal nerve by MRI. The pathogenesis, other causes for TN, and significance of MRI findings have been discussed in Chapters 3 and 5 and are further discussed in Chapter 18.

10.3.2 Indications

1. Classical TN with MRI evidence of NVC.
2. No significant medical comorbidities.

10.3.3 Operative procedures

The technique of MVD for TN is well established and the main features are outlined in fig. 10.2. After the patient undergoes general anaesthetic, and appropriate evoked potential monitoring (brainstem auditory evoked responses) used by some neurosurgeons, the head is turned away from the side of the pain, and the retrosigmoid area is prepared and draped. An incision is made several finger breadths behind the ear, and the skin and muscle are opened. A small craniectomy abutting the transverse and sigmoid sinuses is fashioned. The dura is opened, and the cerebellum may be gently retracted. Under high-power microscopic visualization, the trigeminal nerve is identified, and then the compressive vessel is mobilized from the nerve. Generally, an inert positional graft is then interposed between the compressive vessel and nerve. Once complete, the dura is closed, the craniectomy is reconstituted with a bone substitute, and the muscle and skin are closed. Patients typically are discharged on the third postoperative day and may return to work from 3 to 6 weeks later, depending on the demands of their job.

10.3.3 Outcomes

The major outcomes are shown in fig. 10.3. These include the pain relief periods which are based on reports using the Kaplan–Meier methodology.

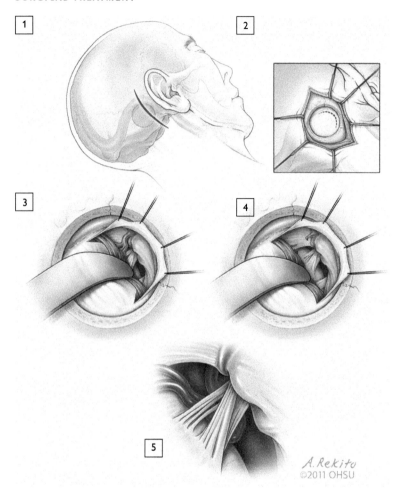

Figure 10.2 Stages of MVD procedure

1 Incision 2 bone exposure 3 exposure of trigeminal nerve and vessels 4 mobilisation 5 trigeminal nerve decompressed

Note use of an infratentorial supracerebellar trajectory to avoid stretching of VII and VIII cranial nerve complex

Complications from this procedure are relatively uncommon, but include ipsilateral hearing loss, other cranial nerve palsies, cerebrospinal fluid leak, and rare infections. Stroke or death from an MVD is exceedingly rare. Many are complications are transient.

CHAPTER 10

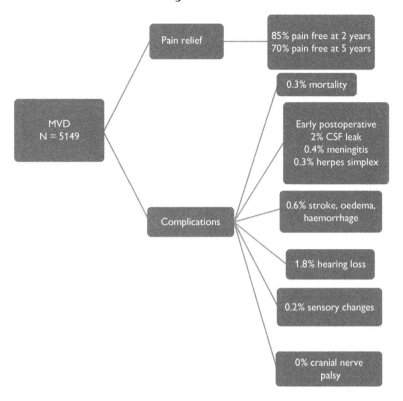

Figure 10.3 Outcomes after MVD
CSF, cerebrospinal fluid.

10.3.3 Predictors of success with MVD for TN

The surgical outcome data to support the use of MVD in certain patients are robust. However, there are clear disparities in outcomes between patients with different types of TN. For example, Miller and colleagues showed that the outcome from MVD was highly correlated with the historical preponderance of lancinating pain. Furthermore, in 2003 patients who underwent MVD for 'typical TN' and 672 patients who underwent MVD for 'atypical TN', the proportions of patients who were free of facial pain at last long-term follow-up (NB: more than one-half of patients were followed for >5 years) were 73.7% and 34.7% in the typical and atypical groups, respectively. The stark difference in outcomes between 'classical' (episodic, lancinating, electrical pain) and 'atypical' (concomitant pain) TN strongly supports the concept that the principal determinant of outcome from MVD is the nature of the pain presentation.

TN type, response to specific medications (i.e. carbamazepine and oxcarbazepine), and presence and severity of NVC utilizing preoperative MRI are established predictors of a positive surgical outcome following MVD. More recent work has focused on the significance of degree of NVC in patients with TN (see Chapters 5 and 6). When the degree of vascular compression is rated on a three-point radiographic grading scale, it therefore seems that grade 1 NVC (contact) is not associated with TN, but grades 2 (compression) and 3 (distortion), are highly correlated with the symptomatic side. The probability of long-term complete pain relief without medications established on a Kaplan–Meier statistical study at 15 years, was demonstrated to be dependent on the grade of compression of the NVC. In grade III, complete relief was achieved in 85%, 73% in grade II, and in grade I, full relief occurred in only 65%.

Retrospective studies that have compared MVD to SRS show that MVD provides higher-quality and more lasting pain relief than SRS.

10.4 Stereotactic radiosurgery

10.4.1 Introduction

The use of SRS for TN began in the early 1990s after the publication of a retrospective international multicentric study. The term Gamma Knife and Cyber Knife are trade names. Since then, SRS has become one of the major neurosurgical approaches for intractable TN. The highest level of evidence is from a single prospective trial demonstrating, in 110 patients, evaluated by independent neurologists, the good safety efficacy with a follow-up of at least 1 year. No prospective trial comparing SRS to other surgical option(s) exists. Retrospective analyses of the literature have clearly shown that SRS was the least invasive of the neurosurgical procedure and has the lowest rate of complication. The long-term follow-up have been studied in three Gamma Knife large cohorts.

10.4.2 Indications

Any patient with TN classical, idiopathic, and secondary to multiple sclerosis (MS). There are no exclusions.

10.4.3 Operative techniques

The vast majority of the papers published on the topic of SRS for TN are based on Gamma Knife radiosurgery. Typically, the stereotactic frame is fixed under local anaesthesia (fig. 10.4).

Stereotactic imaging is performed (MRI +/− computer tomography). Several targets have been described, namely the dorsal root entry zone (DREZ), the plexus triangularis, and the retrogasserian one. The DREZ target has been progressively abandoned, due to a high rate of hypaesthesia and lower long-term efficacy, by moving the isocentre anteriorly in the vast majority of centres, as shown in fig. 10.5.

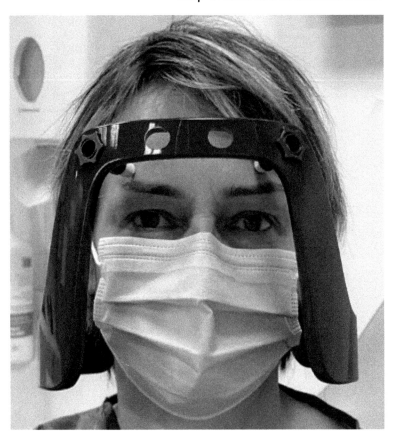

Figure 10.4 SRS headframe

The current retrogasserian target is on the cisternal portion of the trigeminal nerve, 7–8 mm anteriorly to the nerve entrance in the brainstem. The dose prescribed at the 100% is 80–90 Gy depending on the individual anatomy. Lower doses carry a higher rate of failure. Due to the critical target location (close to brainstem) and unique collimator, attention must be paid to the SRS's neuroimaging quality control.

10.4.4 Outcomes

With SRS at the current state of the art, around 90–95% of patients observe pain cessation with a mean delay of 1 month. However, as early as 2 weeks, half the patients are already pain free. The only complication is hypaesthesia occurring

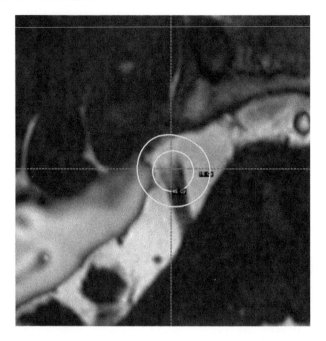

Figure 10.5 Planning MRI

in the 5 years following SRS, which is very bothersome in only 0.6% of patients (fig. 10.6). The later onset of sensory change can be a disappointment in patients who thought they had no complications. Exceptional cases of dry eye have been reported in the past when the DREZ target was used.

Long-term remission

Ten years after SRS, 40–50% of patients are still pain free without medication, while an additional 30% have requested new surgery and the rest are back under medication without new surgery.

10.4.5 Predictors of outcome after SRS

Young patients with typical TN, early SRS, higher prescription dose, and retrogasserian target have been reported to be associated with a higher chance of pain cessation. MS and previous failed MVD decreases the chances of pain cessation after SRS but not megadolicho basilary artery compression. The risk of hypaesthesia is higher when larger volume of nerve is exposed to radiation (Flickinger effect) and when the isocentre is placed at the DREZ or close to it. The biologically effective dose has been recently reported as more predictive

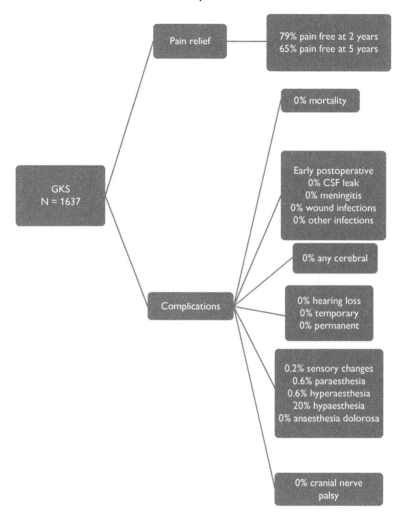

Figure 10.6 Outcomes after SRS
CSF, cerebrospinal fluid; GKS, Gamma Knife surgery.

than physical dose to predict safety and efficacy. The incidence of hypaesthesia is lower than 5% for a biologically effective dose inferior to 1800 Gy and reaches 42% after 2600 Gy.

SRS can be repeated specifically when the patient has been pain free for long years after the first SRS, has developed no hypaesthesia, and does not have other satisfactory therapeutic options. Classically, after primary failure of SRS it is not recommended to repeat SRS.

Due to its minimal invasiveness and because it is the neurosurgical option with the lowest risk, it is frequently the first patient preference.

10.4.6 Role of SRS in patients with MS

Efficacy of SRS in MS is clearly lower compared to the one achieved in classical TN. However, the safety efficacy balance of SRS for TN in MS is comparing favourably to alternatives. Thus, SRS is a very good first-line surgical alternative for treating MS-related TN.

10.5 Percutaneous/ablative procedures

10.5.1 Injection procedures

There are three alternative percutaneous injection procedures:

1. Radiofrequency thermocoagulation (TC).
2. Glycerol rhizolysis (GR).
3. Balloon compression (BC).

Each has its unique set of advantages and drawbacks, and some surgeons are more accustomed to using one than another.

10.5.2 Indications

The indications for percutaneous needle procedures include:

1. Patients who are medically unfit for an open operation.
2. Recurrence of pain after a previous procedure, but not suitable for open surgery.
3. Patient preference for a less invasive procedure.
4. TN associated with multiple sclerosis (MS-TN).

Choosing between these percutaneous procedures is largely dependent on patient preference and experience of the operating surgeon. In our practice, TC is avoided in patients with pure first division (V1) pain due to our finding of an increased risk of inducing corneal anaesthesia. All three procedures are suitable to perform as a 'day case', after morning admission, with afternoon discharge.

10.5.3 Operative technique

Percutaneous procedures are performed under brief general anaesthesia or sedation with fluoroscopic guidance. The operating set-up is shown in fig. 10.7.

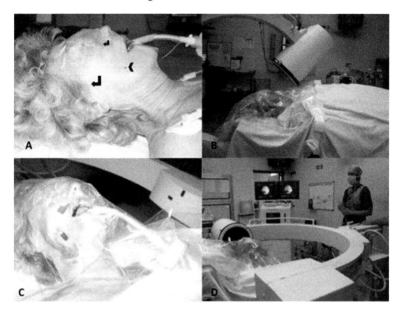

Figure 10.7 Patient undergoing percutaneous procedure

Right-sided balloon compression under general anaesthesia. Note pre-operative procedure side marker is discreetly visible below ear. (A) Arrowhead indicates entry point; smaller angled arrow points towards angled sagittal plane, heavier one towards angled coronal plane for triangulation to trajectory. (B) Image intensifier in place for view along trajectory. (C) Needle in position, image intensifier position for later view of needle/balloon. (D) Balloon catheter entering needle with depth-limiting tape visible against black image intensifier, the screen showing inflated balloon, as in figure 10.8 E.

For GR, a 20-gauge spinal needle is inserted into the medial *foramen ovale* following Härtel's technique, and advanced deep toward the clivus on a lateral projection (fig. 10.7A for landmarks and fig. 10.8 for radiology). After reversal of general anaesthesia, contrast is injected with the patient in the sitting position and head flexed forwards (fig. 10.8F); contrast is then allowed to drip out and is slowly replaced with warmed glycerol (0.36 mL, which is the median volume of Meckel's cave). After subsequent withdrawal of the needle, the patient's position is maintained for at least 2 hours to prevent leakage prior to tissue fixing, which can cause damage to other nerves or chemical meningitis.

For TC, a similar needle insertion technique as for GR is used while the patient is under general anaesthesia, with the needle tip placed further laterally in the *foramen ovale* to reach the trigeminal ganglion, with depth determined by the division selected (fig. 10.8A–C). The electrode tip position is then confirmed by awake testing for evoked paraesthesiae and adjusted if necessary, before re-sedation and heating the electrode to between 65°C and 70°C for 60 seconds. One thermal

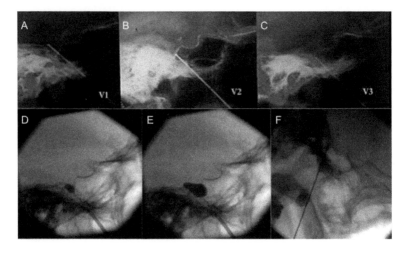

Figure 10.8 Radiological imaging of percutaneous neuroablative procedures

Supine lateral radiographs. **Thermocoagulation (TC).** (A) TC electrode traversing the foramen ovale, the tip reaching just beyond clival line for V1. (B) Electrode tip reaches the clival line for V2. (C) Electrode tip short of clival line, but beyond middle fossa base for V3. **Balloon compression (BC)** (D) Larger needle showing balloon test inflation. (E) Full inflation demonstrating pear shape. **Glycerol rhizolysis (GR).** (F) Erect lateral radiograph with glycerol retained in Meckel's cave around needle tip.

lesion is typically made, except where there is V2 and V3 neuralgia with evoked paraesthesiae in only one of these divisions, in which case a second lesion can be performed for the other division following needle adjustment and retesting. As an alternative, a curved Tew electrode can be utilised to produce a retrogasserian lesion in the nerve root, aiming to limit regeneration for a longer effect.

For BC, following the same needle insertion technique via the middle of the *foramen ovale* on its posterior rim, with a soft Fogarty balloon and minor test inflation with contrast to confirm correct balloon configuration, trigeminal nerve compression entails balloon inflation with 0.35–0.50 mL of contrast to obtain a 'pear' or 'dumbbell' shape (known to improve pain outcomes and reduce complications), with our preference being for three alternating cycles of 60 seconds of inflation and 60 seconds of deflation as shown in fig. 10.7 and fig. 10.8D and E.

10.5.4 Outcomes

The pain relief rates for percutaneous surgery for TN are more variable than for MVD and are influenced by both surgical technique and patient factors. Various studies report excellent initial pain relief in 59–91% of patients after GR, 80–100% after TC, and 82–91% after BC. These results are consistent with our data in which GR and BC produced Barrow Neurological Institute (BNI) class I or II (pain free either without or with medication) pain scores in 63% and 85% respectively;

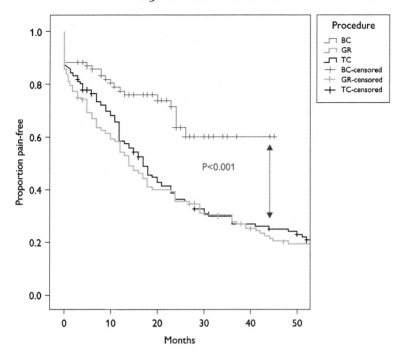

Figure 10.9 Kaplan–Meier analysis of long-term outcomes

Data from a large single-centre retrospective analysis of 393 procedures on 210 TN patients. BC provides significantly longer pain relief than TC and GR (TC and GR give equivalent outcomes as shown by the overlapping KM curves even up to 50 months here), with the surgical technique employed in this study (P < 0.001, log-rank test).

our study reporting a lower TC initial pain-free rate (63%) compared with other studies may reflect the cautious technique (with a single thermal lesion) employed, knowing that the lesion could be repeated in the event of recurrence. Long-term outcomes from these injection procedures in TN from a large retrospective analysis are shown in fig. 10.9.

Regarding BC, the results vary from a median recurrence time of 15.5 to 29 months. The technique for BC varies between studies, and the relatively high durability of relief from BC we have observed (median recurrence time of 24.0 months) may be partly due to the prolonged compression we employed, with three cycles of compression rather than one. Importantly, outcomes and complications from the three procedures are shown in fig. 10.10.

10.5.5 Outcomes in patients with MS and TN

There is limited literature on TC in MS-TN. Pooled analysis of studies suggests a median recurrence time of 27 months, the same as reported in our recent series.

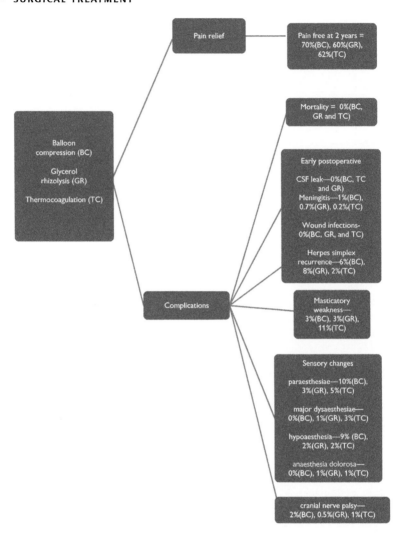

Figure 10.10 Outcomes after ablative procedures

Sensory changes after thermocoagulation are dependent on the intensity of the thermocoagulation.

Moreover, our results from a comparatively large number of procedures in a single centre suggest that TC gives equally long durability of relief in MS-TN as compared with idiopathic TN.

For GR, the reported durability of pain relief in MS-TN is wide-ranging: a median time to recurrence of 17–20 months in three series of 56 patients. A recent systematic review analysed durability of relief from 181 MS-TN patients from combined studies, suggesting a median recurrence time of 12 months for GR but other studies give medians of 20 months. Studies have been conflicting as to whether GR gives worse outcomes in MS-TN than idiopathic TN. Although some studies suggest results from this procedure are similar in the two cohorts, others found a 40% recurrence rate in 34 MS-TN patients at 24 months compared with only 10% in 252 idiopathic TN patients.

We observed that BC provided equally durable relief in MS-TN as in idiopathic TN patients.

10.5.6 Complications

Complications after percutaneous procedures for TN include paraesthesiae and dysaesthesiae, dense facial numbness, corneal anaesthesia, and pterygoid muscle weakness. Less common complications include meningitis, intraoperative cardio-vascular changes (including cardiac standstill), and anaesthesia dolorosa.

Facial numbness is expected to occur after percutaneous TN surgery. A correlation between sensory loss and pain relief following destructive procedures for TN has been suggested, which would explain more destructive lesions giving more durable relief. In line with this, we have observed that postoperative numbness is a significant predictor of favourable outcome for percutaneous procedures, and moreover is a significant predictor for lack of recurrence on long-term follow-up. In our experience, patients usually tolerate a degree of numbness and/or sensory disturbance postoperatively if they achieve adequate pain relief from TN, and should be preoperatively counselled for this. The technique we employ for BC, with three cycles of 60 seconds of BC, is likely to have a stronger destructive effect than a single cycle of compression reported in some studies, explaining the higher degree of postoperative numbness compared with GR and TC we have observed.

10.6 Other posterior fossa procedures

Although the incidence of this practice is not clearly presented in the literature, some neurosurgeons have effectively confounded the results of MVD with the addition of unintentional, and intentional, surgical trauma to the nerve in the form of 'massage', or even more aggressive forms of neurolysis in combination with MVD. Adams has, in fact, previously suggested that 'the basis of MVD could be trauma to the nerve during the operative exposure and "decompression"'. Further, it is known that internal neurolysis can have a profound effect on eliminating TN, to a degree that is surprisingly comparable to the results from MVD.

It is conceivable that what has been reported as the outcome of MVD has been, in many instances, the outcome of a hybrid procedure of MVD and neurolysis.

Prior to high-quality MRIs, neurosurgeons would enter the posterior fossa and find no NVC. In these cases, a partial sensory rhizotomy would be done. Both partial sensory rhizotomy and internal neurolysis can result in comparable pain relief periods to MVD but patients will report significant sensory loss in potentially all three divisions.

10.7 Other procedures

There is no high-quality evidence for any of the procedures shown in fig. 10.11. Many of them are peripheral techniques and so can be carried out under local anaesthesia in patients with significant medical comorbidities and provide on average less than 1 year of pain relief. They are linked with fewer complications.

10.8 Decision-making

There is an increasing need for shared decision-making in order to ensure personalized care. 'Personalised care means people have choice and control over the way their care is planned and delivered, based on "what matters" to them and their individual strengths and needs' (https://www.england.nhs.uk/publicat ion/shared-decision-making-summary-guide/). This is especially important in TN when there is a significant range of options with variable outcomes and associated risks. Patients' quality of life, ability to carry out activities of daily living, and mood need to be taken into account when deciding on surgical options including highlighting that even though pain relief may be achieved, complications can have a significant impact on other outcomes.

Which surgical procedures should the two patients described in Table 10.1 and Table 10.2 have and how could the patients be helped in making their decisions? Their TN is not only resulting in severe pain but is having a significant impact on their quality of life.

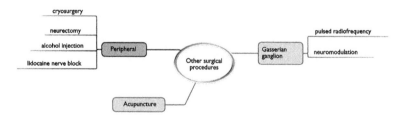

Figure 10.11 Other surgical procedures

Table 10.1 Patient scenario 1	
Features	Surgical choice of procedure
Sex, age	Male, 58 years
History of pain	8-year history of classical TN with MRI evidence of NVC. Right-sided V2 and V3. Remission periods getting shorter and each relapse getting more intense with increased frequency. Has used high-dose carbamazepine and now on oxcarbazepine 1500 mg. No comorbidities but is worried about having major surgery
Effect of pain on lifestyle	Interferes with work and has had to take time off work

Table 10.2 Patient scenario 2	
Features	Surgical management with medical comorbidities
Sex, age	Female, 80 years
History of pain	19-year history of classical TN, right third division, periods of severe pain 2–3 weeks and then remission periods of years but more recently only 1–2 months. Carbamazepine maximum 800 mg controls the pain but results in severe side effects at the higher doses. Only used phenytoin in the past
Current episode	Began 1½ years ago, no remission since. Now getting worse and attacks of pain every hour. No longer controlled on carbamazepine 800 mg, cognitive impairment, tiredness
Medical history	Left hemi-glossectomy and neck dissection 5 years ago, bilateral hip replacements, atrial fibrillation, and has a pacemaker
Current other medications	Warfarin, antihypertensives, statin

Patient 1 could have any of the options described in this chapter. He has understandably got concerns about major surgery, that is, MVD, which potentially is his best long-term option. He would benefit from a face-to-face discussion with both a neurosurgeon and physician being present at the same consultation. His concerns need to be identified and evidence provided. We have found that a joint clinic with a neurosurgeon and a physician being present at the same time enables the patient and their significant other to ask questions and get opinions from both experts. A patient service evaluation of such a clinic has shown high satisfaction on the part of the patients. Providing him with a decision guide such

Ottawa Personal Decision Guide
For People Making Health or Social Decisions

❶ Clarify your decision.

What decision do you face?

What are your reasons for making this decision?

When do you need to make a choice?

How far along are you with making a choice?	Not thought about it	Close to choosing
	Thinking about it	Made a choice

❷ Explore your decision.

Knowledge	**Values**	**Certainty**
List the options and benefits and risks you know.	Rate each benefit and risk using stars (★) to show how much each one matters to you.	Choose the option with the benefits that matter most to you. Avoid the options with the risks that matter most to you.

	Reasons to Choose this Option Benefits / Advantages / Pros	How much it matters to you: 0★ not at all 5★ a great deal	Reasons to Avoid this Option Risks / Disadvantages / Cons	How much it matters to you: 0★ not at all 5★ a great deal
Option #1				
Option #2				
Option #3				

Which option do you prefer?	Option #1	Option #2	Option #3	Unsure

Support

Who else is involved?			
Which option do they prefer?			
Is this person pressuring you?	Yes No	Yes No	Yes No
How can they support you?			

What role do you prefer in making the choice?	Share the decision with… Decide myself after hearing views of… Someone else decides…

Figure 10.12 Decision aid

Available at: https://decisionaid.ohri.ca/decguide.html

You may use any of these guides without requesting permission. These guides are protected by copyright but are freely available for you to use, provided you: a) cite the reference in any documents or publications; b) do not charge for or profit from them; and c) do not alter them except for prefilling them for a specific condition/decision as necessary.

⊙ Identify your decision making needs.

Adapted from The SURE Test © 2008 O'Connor & Légaré.

Knowledge	Do you know the benefits and risks of each option?	Yes	No
Values	Are you clear about which benefits and risks matter most to you?	Yes	No
Support	Do you have enough support and advice to make a choice?	Yes	No
Certainty	Do you feel sure about the best choice for you?	Yes	No

If you answer 'no' to any question, you can work through steps two ⊙ and four ⊙, focusing on your needs.
People who answer "No" to one or more of these questions are more likely to delay their decision, change their mind, feel regret about their choice or blame others for bad outcomes.

⊙ Plan the next steps based on your needs.

Decision making needs	✓ Things you could try
Knowledge If you feel you do NOT have enough facts	Find out more about the options and the chances of the benefits and risks. List your questions. List where to find the answers (e.g. library, health professionals, counsellors):
Values If you are NOT sure which benefits and risks matter most to you	Review the stars in step two ⊙ to see what matters most to you. Find people who know what it is like to experience the benefits and risks. Talk to others who have made the decision. Read stories of what mattered most to others. Discuss with others what matters most to you.
Support If you feel you do NOT have enough support If you feel PRESSURE from others to make a specific choice	Discuss your options with a trusted person (e.g. health professional, counsellor, family, friends). Find help to support your choice (e.g. funds, transport, child care). Focus on the views of others who matter most. Share your guide with others. Ask others to fill in this guide. (See where you agree. If you disagree on facts, get more information. If you disagree on what matters most, consider the other person's views. Take turns to listen to what the other person says matters most to them.) Find a person to help you and others involved.
Certainty If you feel UNSURE about the best choice for you Other factors making the decision DIFFICULT	Work through steps two ⊙ and four ⊙, focusing on your needs. List anything else you could try:

Ottawa Personal Decision Guide © 2015 O'Connor, Stacey, Jacobsen. Ottawa Hospital Research Institute & University of Ottawa, Canada.   Page 2 of 2

Figure 10.12 Continued

Table 10.3 Patient scenario 3

Features	Surgical recurrence
Sex, age	Male, 41 years
History of pain	15 years ago TN right V2 only, responded to carbamazepine but significant side effects. Had radiofrequency thermocoagulation 11 years ago complete pain relief, has numbness including decreased corneal reflex. Pain recurred year ago
Location and radiation	Right V1 and V2
Characteristics of pain	Paroxysmal, each attack several seconds; occurring intermittently every few hours
Severity/character	Very severe, sharp electric shock, shooting
Provoking factors	Washing, brushing hair, cold wind
Relieving factors	Carbamazepine 1600 mg, gabapentin 300 mg not controlling the pain
Associated factors	Numbness, intermittent redness of the cheek
Effect of pain on lifestyle	Cannot work as a postman, taken 2 weeks off, mild depression
Examination	Slight numbness only V2 and V3, poor oral hygiene on right side MRI no compression

as the Ottawa Decision Aid with his options listed (https://decisionaid.ohri.ca/decguide.html) (fig. 10.12) would allow him to discuss further the pros and cons with significant others and other patients who have undergone the procedure (see Chapter 17).

Patient 2 has multiple medical comorbidities which make both medical and surgical treatments difficult. Certainly, a MVD is not a possibility. Percutaneous/ablative surgery which involves penetration through the foramen ovale may be risky given her cardiac history and use of anticoagulants. Potentially her best option would be SRS as it is the least invasive. However, it can take some weeks for SRS to become effective so she may need some short-term changes to her medications (e.g. addition of lamotrigine to provide better pain control).

Patient 3 (Table 10.3) had successful surgery in the past but has now had a recurrence and it is no longer controlled by medications. Which surgical procedure should he have?

Table 10.4 Patient scenario 4

Features	Secondary TN post surgery
Sex, age	Female, 61 years
History	10 years ago excision of left acoustic neuroma, symptom at the time of hearing loss. 2 years later develops TN left all three divisions. Relapses and remissions and managed on antiepileptics. 1 year ago required admission due to severity of pain and dehydration. Eventually controlled on drugs. Now presents with severe pain taking carbamazepine 1600 mg, gabapentin 1500 mg. Classic TN symptoms MRI shows NVC of the trigeminal nerve. No evidence of recurrence of acoustic neuroma
Effect of pain on lifestyle	Poor mood, unable to work
Examination	No sensory changes

Given that there is some residual numbness, there is an increased risk of causing more numbness and potential anaesthesia dolorosa when doing percutaneous lesion. The option would potentially be SRS as it has the lowest rate of sensory deficit.

Patient 4 (Table 10.4) presents with a difficult problem and several options may be proposed. This may be dependent on the centre which is treating the patient.

10.9 Lay summary

There are a range of surgical treatments that patients can undergo if medical therapies are no longer effective and quality of life is impaired. The most invasive procedure is a major neurosurgical procedure, MVD, which is suitable for patients with NVC and who are medically fit. It provides the longest pain-free period and least long-term complications. Of the ablative procedures, SRS is the least invasive procedure with the lowest chance of causing significant sensory loss. All these procedures on average give a few years of pain relief and can be repeated. Pain relief is often proportional to degree of postoperative numbness which may impact quality of life. Patients need to discuss the various surgical options with both their healthcare providers and their significant others in order to make the best choice. Table 10.5 summarizes the outcomes from the major surgical procedures discussed in this chapter; the percentages do vary in different reports and this table attempts to present the best evidence we have at present.

Table 10.5 Summary of outcomes for all procedures in percentages

Outcome	MVD N = 5149	SRS N = 1168	TC N = 4533	BC N = 755	GR N = 289
Pain free 2 years	85	79	62	70	60
Pain free 5 years	70	65	20	50	20
Deaths	0.3	0	0	0	0
Cerebrospinal fluid leak	2	0	0	0	0
Meningitis	0.4	0	0.02–0.2	1–5.7	0–0.7
Stroke haemorrhage, swelling (oedema)	0.6	0	0	0	0
Hearing loss	1.8	0	0–0.1	0	0–0.3
Other nerve involvement	4	0.2	0–0.8	0–1.6	0
Herpes simplex postoperative	0.3	0	0–2	0–6	0–8
Eye infection (keratitis)	0	0.3	0–1.2	0–0.1	0
Eye numbness (corneal hypaesthesia)	0.3	0	6.6	0.7	6.6
Weakness of eating muscles	0	0	6.2–11	3–4.5	1.7–3
Face mild numbness (hyperaesthesia, paraesthesia)	2.9	15.8–20	5–18.8	10–14.6	3–39.8
Face moderate numbness (dysaesthesia)	0.02	0–0.6	3	0	1
Severe numbness (anaesthesia dolorosa)	0.02	0	0.6–1	0–0.1	0.7–1

It is extremely difficult to compare the different techniques as the number of patients involved is very variable. Pain-free periods are recorded very differently. The results presented are based on the published guidelines and other reports in the literature, but all are low-grade evidence.

BC, balloon compression; GR glycerol rhizolysis; MVD, microvascular decompression; SRS, stereotactic radiosurgery; TC, radiofrequency thermocoagulation.

10.10 RECOMMENDED READING

Akram H, Mirza B, Kitchen N, et al. Proposal for evaluating the quality of reports of surgical interventions in the treatment of trigeminal neuralgia: the Surgical Trigeminal Neuralgia Score. Neurosurg Focus. 2013;35:E3. doi: 10.3171/2013.6.FOCUS13213

Barzaghi LR, Albano L, Scudieri C, et al. Factors affecting long-lasting pain relief after Gamma Knife radiosurgery for trigeminal neuralgia: a single institutional analysis and literature review. Neurosurg Rev. 2021;44:2797–808. doi: 10.1007/s10143-021-01474-9

Brînzeu A, Drogba L, Sindou M. Reliability of MRI for predicting characteristics of neurovascular conflicts in trigeminal neuralgia: implications for surgical decision making. J Neurosurg. 2018;130:611–21. doi: 10.3171/2017.8JNS171222

Noorani I, Lodge A, Vajramani G, et al. Comparing percutaneous treatments of trigeminal neuralgia: 19 years of experience in a single centre. Stereotact Funct Neurosurg. 2016;94:75–85. doi: 10.1159/000445077

Noorani I, Lodge A, Vajramani G, et al. The effectiveness of percutaneous balloon compression, thermocoagulation, and glycerol rhizolysis for trigeminal neuralgia in multiple sclerosis. Neurosurgery. 2019;85:E684–92. doi: 10.1093/neuros/nyz103

Regis J, Tuleasca C. Fifteen years of Gamma Knife surgery for trigeminal neuralgia in the Journal of Neurosurgery: history of a revolution in functional neurosurgery. J Neurosurg. 2011;115 Suppl:2–7. doi: 10.3171/2011.12.GKS

Sindou M, Brinzeu A. Topography of the pain in classical trigeminal neuralgia: insights into somatotopic organization. Brain. 2020;143:531–40. doi: 10.1093/brain/awz407.

Taha JM, Tew JM Jr, Buncher CR. A prospective 15-year follow up of 154 consecutive patients with trigeminal neuralgia treated by percutaneous stereotactic radiofrequency thermal rhizotomy. J Neurosurg. 1995;83:989–93. doi: 10.3171/jns.1995.83.6.0989

Tuleasca C, Carron R, Resseguier N, et al. Decreased probability of initial pain cessation in classic trigeminal neuralgia treated with gamma knife surgery in case of previous microvascular decompression: a prospective series of 45 patients with >1 year of follow-up. Neurosurgery. 2015;77:87–94. doi:10.1227/neu.0000000000000739

Tuleasca C, Paddick I, Hopewell JW, et al. Establishment of a therapeutic ratio for gamma knife radiosurgery of trigeminal neuralgia: the critical importance of biologically effective dose versus physical dose. World Neurosurg. 2019;134:e204–13. doi:10.1016/j.wneu.2019.10.021

Tuleasca C, Régis J, Sahgal A, et al. Stereotactic radiosurgery for trigeminal neuralgia: a systematic review. J Neurosurg. 2018;27:1–25. Doi 10.3171/2017.9.JNS17545

More surgical details can be found in textbooks such as Jannetta PJ, editor. Trigeminal Neuralgia. Oxford: Oxford University Press; 2011. ISBN 9780195342833.

10.11 Continuing professional development

1. Which of the surgical procedures is least likely to result in no sensory loss and longest pain-free period?
2. Which of the following statements are true?
   a. There is a randomized controlled trial comparing MVD and SRS.

b. Percutaneous/ablative procedures are suitable for patients with medical comorbidities.

c. SRS is suitable for patients with MS.

d. The average pain relief period for MVD is 2 years.

3. How may healthcare professionals help patients make a decision about which surgical procedure to undergo?

Painful trigeminal neuropathy

Satu K. Jääskeläinen and Turo Nurmikko

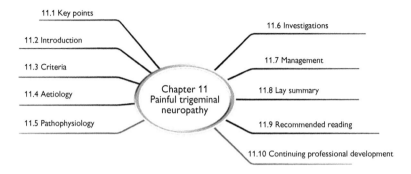

Figure 11.1 Plan of chapter

11.1 KEY POINTS

1. Painful trigeminal neuropathy (PTN) is defined as pain lasting over 3 months and occurring within 6 months after any type of damage on the nerve or its central pathways.
2. Causes include iatrogenic and other injuries, tumours, infection, stroke, and systemic disease (e.g. diabetes, hypothyroidism, and connective tissue disorder).
3. The main characteristics of PTN are sensory deficits combined with ongoing pain that may fluctuate in intensity.
4. Gain-of-function signs and brief electric-shock like pains may be reported but they are not the main feature—an important distinction from trigeminal neuralgia.
5. With time, both the sensory signs and pain may spread outside the primarily affected division(s)—extra-segmentally and even over the midline.
6. The degree of certainty for the diagnosis of PTN depends on history and symptoms (possible), unambiguous clinical signs (probable), or abnormalities in specific investigations (psychophysical, neurophysiological, biopsy, and structural imaging) (definite).
7. The treatment is similar to that of neuropathic pain in general, with pharmacotherapy as the first-line, and novel therapeutic neuromodulation techniques (repetitive transcranial magnetic stimulation, transcranial direct current stimulation) as the second-line options.
8. In chronic PTN, psychiatric comorbidity is common, and multidisciplinary psychosocial treatment advised.

11.2 Introduction

Table 11.1 provides details of a patient with a painful trigeminal neuropathy (PTN).

11.3 Description, classification, and diagnostic criteria

Painful trigeminal pain conditions comprise facial or oral pain in the distribution of one or more branches of the trigeminal nerve, uni- or bilaterally, with indications of neural damage, and duration of at least 3 months. The primary pain is usually continuous or near-continuous, but may fluctuate in intensity. It is commonly described as burning, squeezing, or aching, with paraesthesia ('pins and needles'). Superimposed brief pain paroxysms may occur but they are not the predominant pain type distinguishing PTN from trigeminal neuralgia.

In the International Classification of Headache Disorders, third edition (ICHD-3), post-traumatic and other PTNs are listed under the heading '13.1.2 Painful trigeminal neuropathy'. More recently, the first edition of the International Classification of Orofacial Pain (ICOP-I) has further developed the classification of orofacial pain including PTN, or trigeminal neuropathic pain, under the heading 4.1.2, see Table 11.2. Both classifications necessitate clinical sensory signs: either loss or gain of function. ICOP-I requests additional confirmatory test results for the diagnosis, otherwise PTN will remain probable.

The main symptoms and findings in PTN consist of loss of function, hypoaesthesia, or anaesthesia, in one or more sensory modalities within one or more trigeminal distributions, with pain onset within 6 months of a known causal nerve damage, and frequently, positive sensory signs, as in other neuropathic pain conditions. Likewise, PTN may show lancinating or brief, electric shock-like pains, especially when there is a causal space-occupying lesion producing focal demyelination of the large myelinated fibres. Combined with loss-of-function signs, the patients may demonstrate gain-of-function symptoms such as paraesthesia, allodynia, hyperaesthesia, or dysaesthesia, and positive wind-up of pain to repeated stimulation. In PTN, with time, both the pain and the sensory signs may spread from the original to neighbouring intact distributions, or bilaterally over the midline.

Like neuropathic pain in general, PTN diagnosis can be defined as 'possible', 'probable', or 'definite' according to increasing levels of evidence from clinical history and signs up to confirmatory results from psychophysical and neurophysiological tests or imaging studies. In the ICOP-I, this likelihood has been adopted in the classification system with a separate subclass 'probable' for each entity with only clinical evidence, while the diagnosis proper demands confirmatory test evidence and is thus compatible with 'definite' PTN.

11.4 Aetiology

The commonest cause of PTN is injury to the nerve, either from a medical, surgical, or dental procedure, or a less specific mechanical, thermal, chemical, or

Table 11.1 Patient scenario I

Features	Scenario
Sex, age	Male, 53 years
Location and radiation	Left V2, maximum pain area around upper incisor
Characteristics	Continuous, fluctuating, no paroxysms; associated with subjective numbness of left cheek
Severity and quality of pain	Moderate to severe in intensity; burning and smarting
Provoking factors	Mechanical static pressure over the painful site
Relieving factors	Minimal benefit from tramadol and gabapentinoids, but intolerable side effects. rTMS has produced significant pain reduction for 6 months, long-term maintenance therapy at home with portable tDCS device is under consideration
Associated features	Nil
History of pain	16 years ago had multiple dental procedures. Root treatment with complications for left upper incisor, permanent local pain since. Over the years pain slowly expanded to over most of V2 division
Effect of pain on lifestyle and mood	Welder. Finds wearing welding helmet difficult. Works part-time only. Low mood; slightly better after attending an outpatient pain management programme
Clinical examination	Bedside sensory testing (comparison with right mirror image site): reduced sensitivity to heat, cold, pinprick. Reduced mechanical pain pressure threshold
Investigations	Brainstem reflexes: blink reflex responses (R2i and R2c) delayed with stimulation of the left infraorbital nerve (ION) Thermal QST at the left ION distribution: hypoaesthesia to cooling and warming
Diagnosis	Chronic neuropathic pain due to infraorbital nerve injury on the left side, probably associated with previous dental surgical procedures

radiation injury to the head, face, or intraoral structures. If pain and sensory changes develop within 6 months of the event, the condition is called post-traumatic PTN. PTN may also arise from patient-related factors such as vascular anomalies or stroke influencing the trigeminal pathways (e.g. lateral medullary infarction), and space-occupying lesions (tumours, metastases, multiple sclerosis plaque) that compress or invade the trigeminal sensory afferents. In addition, infections (notably, herpes zoster) or systemic diseases (e.g. connective tissue disorders, hypothyroidism, and diabetes) may cause PTN (often with signs of

Table 11.2 Classification

Diagnosis	Definition ICHD-3	Definition ICOP-I
Painful post-traumatic trigeminal neuropathy (ICHD-3) Post-traumatic trigeminal neuropathic pain (ICOP-I)	Unilateral facial or oral pain following and caused by trauma to the trigeminal nerve, within 6 months of injury, with symptoms and clinical signs of trigeminal nerve dysfunction: negative and/or positive signs within the traumatically lesioned distribution(s). Previous name: anaesthesia dolorosa	Pain within the distribution(s) of trigeminal nerve(s), persisting or recurring for >3 months, associated with somatosensory symptoms/signs in the same distribution, onset within 6 months after the injury Definite: confirmed with diagnostic test(s) Probable: not confirmed with diagnostic test(s)
Painful trigeminal neuropathy attributed to other disorder (ICHD-3) Trigeminal neuropathic pain attributed to other disorder (ICOP-I)	Unilateral or bilateral facial or oral pain in the distribution(s) of one or more branches of the trigeminal nerve, caused by a disorder other than an external trauma, but known to be able to cause painful trigeminal neuropathy with clinically evident positive (hyperalgesia, allodynia) and/or negative (hypaesthesia, hypalgesia) signs of trigeminal nerve dysfunction, affecting one or both trigeminal nerves Evidence of causation demonstrated by both of the following: 1. Pain is localized to the distribution(s) of the trigeminal nerve(s) affected by the disorder 2. Pain developed after onset of the disorder, or led to its discovery	Pain, in a neuroanatomically plausible area within the distribution(s) of one or both trigeminal nerve(s), persisting or recurring for >3 months A disorder other than herpes zoster or trauma but known to be capable of causing, and explaining, the trigeminal neuropathic pain, has been diagnosed Pain has developed after onset of the presumed causative disorder, or has led to its discovery Pain is associated with somatosensory symptoms and/or signs in the same neuroanatomically plausible distribution Definite: confirmed with diagnostic test(s) Probable: not confirmed with diagnostic test(s)

Table 11.2 Continued		
Diagnosis	Definition ICHD-3	Definition ICOP-I
Idiopathic painful trigeminal neuropathy (ICHD-3) Idiopathic trigeminal neuropathic pain (ICOP-I)	Unilateral or bilateral pain in the distribution of one or more branches of the trigeminal nerve(s), indicative of neural damage but of unknown aetiology	Unilateral or bilateral facial pain in the distribution(s) of one or more branches of the trigeminal nerve, indicative of neural damage and persisting or recurring for >3 months, but of unknown aetiology Definite: confirmed with diagnostic test(s) Probable: not confirmed with diagnostic test(s)

concomitant polyneuropathy). When no cause can be identified, the condition is called idiopathic PTN (formerly 'neuritis').

11.5 Pathophysiology

Pathophysiological mechanisms of PTN are similar to those in neuropathic pain in general (see also Chapters 5, 6, and 13). A prerequisite is a lesion or disease affecting the somatosensory system either in the peripheral or central nervous system. The type of lesion causing PTN is typically a partial axonal injury, including damage to the small fibre system (A delta and C fibres, or their central pathways). Purely demyelinating neuropathies rarely cause pain, but it may occur, especially in compression neuropathies, with paraesthesia and allodynia.

Certain neurophysiological features of PTN are associated with specific pathophysiological alterations in the trigeminal nerve. The intensity of the characteristic continuous burning pain is correlated with greater deficits in small fibre function, shown, for example, by small amplitudes of pain-evoked potentials (which reflect axonal damage of the small A delta fibre tracts). Paroxysmal pain associates with prolonged blink reflex latencies and slow nerve conduction velocities, a finding compatible with demyelination.

Deficient habituation of the pain-evoked potentials and blink reflex in PTN is compatible with deficient top-down inhibition of the trigeminal brainstem nuclear complex, possibly caused by insufficient activity of the brain dopamine–opioid neurotransmitter system. Non-invasive therapeutic brain stimulation, known to release these endogenous neurotransmitters, may work by boosting the system with resultant pain relief, and simultaneous amelioration of often concomitant depression and anxiety that have been linked to dopamine deficiency.

11.6 Investigations

History and symptoms form the basis in the diagnostic process of PTN. Clinical examination should include standardized sensory testing of several sensory modalities, at least tactile, thermal, and pain sensation. Routine clinical sensory testing is not very reliable after the acute phase of nerve injury: at chronic stages of PTN, the diagnostic sensitivity of qualitative sensory examination can be as low as 0%, depending on the extent and recovery of the original injury. By contrast, including quantitative sensory testing (QST) for detection of sensory deficits in the bed- or chairside examination increases the diagnostic yield significantly. For example, the testing of simple tactile detection threshold increases sensitivity to 60%. Thermal QST, especially warm and cool detection threshold measurement, improves diagnostic accuracy further, also at the chronic stage, whereas thermal pain detection is insensitive. An advantage of QST over other investigations is in its ability to quantify positive sensory signs, such as allodynia and hyperalgesia. Clinical neurophysiological tests, electromyography and neurography, show the highest diagnostic values ranging between 85% and 100% both at the early and late stages of PTN. Furthermore, brainstem reflex recordings, blink and masseter reflex, show high diagnostic accuracy in trigeminal system lesions with sensitivities ranging from 50% to 100%, the highest values reported for trigeminal brainstem lesions. With blink reflex habituation, the efficacy of top-down inhibition of the trigeminal brainstem complex can be measured, which may in the future aid in tailoring pharmacotherapy on individual patient level. Epidermal nerve fibre density (ENFD) measurement from both facial skin and intraoral mucosal biopsies can be used to verify the diagnosis with high accuracy for small fibre damage. Fig. 11.2 shows the relative values of different investigations at early and late stages of trigeminal neuropathy.

Definite diagnosis of PTN requires confirmation with the aid of these confirmatory laboratory investigations that greatly increase the diagnostic accuracy. Thorough neurophysiological investigation, combined with QST, also gives good topography-level diagnosis, which aids in focusing subsequent structural imaging when considered necessary. Magnetic resonance imaging, with contrast enhancement and thin slices of the brainstem, is invaluable in confirming the site and nature of structural involvement of the trigeminal system, especially within the intracranial space, and in cases with neuritis. It should be noted, though, that plain magnetic resonance imaging and computed tomography scans may remain falsely negative even when there is structural involvement of the trigeminal system.

11.7 Evidence-based management

If the cause cannot be removed or acted on (e.g. tumour), the same treatment guidelines apply as for neuropathic pain in general. Medication forms the first-line approach, with best efficacy values (lowest number needed to treat) shown for tricyclic antidepressants, strong opioids, tramadol, and botulinum toxin A, and

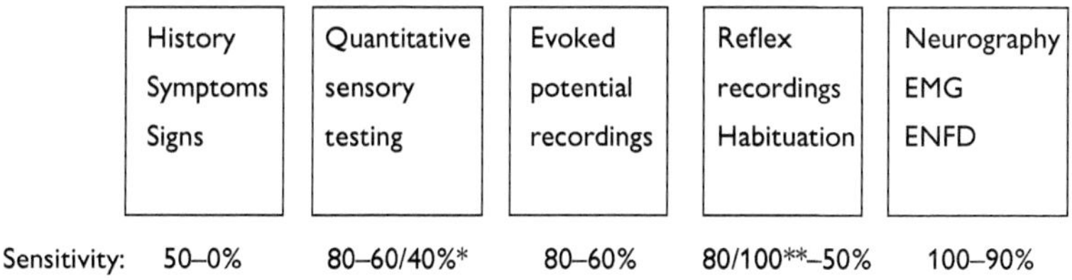

History Symptoms Signs	Quantitative sensory testing	Evoked potential recordings	Reflex recordings Habituation	Neurography EMG ENFD

Sensitivity: 50–0% 80–60/40%* 80–60% 80/100**–50% 100–90%

Figure 11.2 Flow chart of the relative diagnostic sensitivity of different investigations for trigeminal neuropathy

EMG, electromyography; ENFD, epidermal nerve fibre density.

*lowest sensitivity for heat pain detection thresholds, ** highest sensitivities in trigeminal brainstem lesions

modest efficacy for serotonin–noradrenaline reuptake inhibitors, pregabalin, and gabapentin. Fig. 11.3 summarizes pharmacotherapeutic options for the treatment of PTN. For intraoral pain in primary burning mouth syndrome, caused in the majority of patients by focal small fibre neuropathy, there is additional evidence for efficacy of topical clonazepam treatment. Acute ophthalmic herpes zoster needs early aggressive antiviral treatment, and an ophthalmic consultation. Involvement of second and third divisions is rare. For trigeminal postherpetic neuralgia, the same medical treatment applies as in PTN in general but treatment with capsaicin 8% patch requires caution (and in most countries the advice is against its use for facial areas).

If pharmacotherapy fails or adverse effects limit its use, novel non-invasive therapeutic neuromodulation methods offer an alternative with repetitive

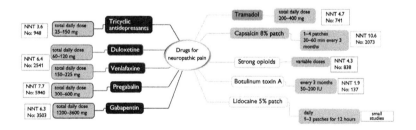

Figure 11.3 Pharmacotherapy

Drugs in black boxes are first line, drugs in grey boxes second line, drugs in white boxes third line

NNT number needed to treat. No, number of patients involved in the trials

Tricyclic antidepressants include: amitriptyline, imipramine, and clomipramine not > 75 mg/day in elderly (> 65 years). No evidence to support use of opioids in trigeminal neuropathic pain

transcranial magnetic stimulation (rTMS) and transcranial direct current stimulation (tDCS). These brain stimulation techniques seem to be most efficient for neuropathic pain within the trigeminal distribution, including PTN, PHN, burning mouth syndrome, and trigeminal neuralgia. Of note, there is currently A level evidence for efficacy of rTMS, and B level evidence of tDCS for neuropathic pain in general. The role of invasive neuromodulation techniques (trigeminal nerve stimulation, trigeminal ganglion stimulation, deep brain stimulation) remains uncertain. Small case series suggest some effectiveness but controlled studies are lacking. Neuroablative surgery should be avoided as it poses a risk for worsening rather than relieving pain.

Because of common psychiatric comorbidity in PTN, multidisciplinary psychosocial management is often necessary in addition to analgesic interventions (see Chapter 16).

11.7.1 Clinical tips and future topics

It is important to recognize that with time, pain and sensory deficits of PTN may spread outside the originally affected nerve territory to neighbouring areas, and even bilaterally, as shown in the mental nerve distribution with spreading hypoaesthesia in thermal QST but normal neurography. This evolution of signs makes the differential diagnosis particularly demanding between peripheral PTN or brainstem lesions and persistent idiopathic facial pain (formerly atypical facial pain). Yet, the diagnostic acumen can be improved using clinical neurophysiological and psychophysical testing and ENFD measurement. As a case in point, burning mouth syndrome exemplifies an enigmatic orofacial pain condition in which systematic studies applying specific diagnostic tests have elucidated different neurogenic aetiologies that may coexist: (1) focal small fibre neuropathy of the intraoral mucosa, (2) painful peripheral or central trigeminal system lesion, and (3) deficient top-down inhibition of the trigeminal brainstem complex. Despite growing evidence for neuropathic aetiology in the majority of patients with burning mouth syndrome, current classification systems do not unambiguously recognize it as PTN, or link it to neural mechanisms, although with growing evidence this is likely to happen in the future.

Trigeminal nerve injury may or may not lead to PTN. There is active research looking for, and emerging evidence on, neurophysiological or genetic biomarkers with potential to predict the development of PTN.

11.8 Lay summary

PTN is defined as a neuropathic pain condition affecting the face or oral cavity, and lasting for more than 3 months. Any damage to the trigeminal nerve of the face, or related nerve pathways running in the central nervous system, may cause it and the associated alteration in skin sensitivity. Most commonly it is seen in people who have suffered facial injuries, or undergone dental and surgical procedures, but it may also be encountered in people with systemic disease (e.g.

diabetes, connective tissue disease, hypothyroidism, or widespread peripheral neuropathy). The condition may be diagnosed during routine clinical examination. To confirm the diagnosis, the managing doctor may order specific tests, such as quantitative sensory testing (QST), neurophysiological tests, biopsies from affected skin or mucosa, or magnetic resonance imaging of the head. Pain medication that is recommended for neuropathic pain in general is usually prescribed first. If medication does not help or causes adverse effects, despite dose adjustments, non-invasive brain stimulation with magnetic pulses (rTMS) or weak electric current (tDCS) as novel treatment options could be considered. In long-lasting PTN, depression or anxiety may occur, and should be addressed with appropriate supportive measures.

11.9 RECOMMENDED READING

Finnerup NB, Attal N, Haroutounian S, et al. Pharmacotherapy for neuropathic pain in adults: a systematic review and meta-analysis. Lancet Neurol. 2015;14:162–73. doi: 10.1016/S1474-4422(14)70251-0

Jääskeläinen SK. Differential diagnosis of chronic neuropathic orofacial pain: role of clinical neurophysiology. J Clin Neurophysiol. 2019;36:422–9. doi: 10.1097/WNP.0000000000000583

Jääskeläinen SK, Woda A. Burning mouth syndrome. Cephalalgia. 2017;37:627–47. doi: 10.1177/033310241769488

Lefaucheur JP, Aleman A, Baeken C, et al. Evidence-based guidelines on the therapeutic use of repetitive transcranial magnetic stimulation (rTMS): an update (2014–2018). Clin Neurophysiol. 2020;131:474–528. doi: 10.1016/j.clinph.2019.11.002

Lindholm P, Lamusuo S, Taiminen T, et al. Right secondary somatosensory cortex – a promising novel target for the treatment of drug-resistant neuropathic orofacial pain with repetitive transcranial magnetic stimulation. Pain. 2015;156:1276–83. doi: 10.1097/j.pain.0000000000000175

11.10 Continuing professional development

1. Describe the main differences in the classification of PTN in the ICHD-3 and ICOP-I. How could these classifications help you in clinical practice with orofacial pain patients and scientific research on orofacial pain?

2. How would you proceed with the diagnostic process in a case of a 44-year-old lady with facial pain after extraction of lower wisdom tooth on the right side 3 months ago? How would you treat this patient, if she had post-traumatic PTN?

Glossopharyngeal neuralgia and neuropathy and nervus intermedius neuralgia and neuropathy

Claudia Sommer, Turo Nurmikko, and Raymond F. Sekula Jr

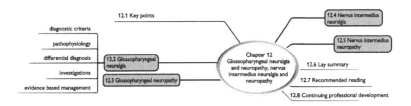

Figure 12.1 Plan of chapter

12.1 KEY POINTS

1. Diagnosis is clinical, based on quality and location of pain; neuroimaging serves to delineate the likely cause.
2. Glossopharyngeal neuralgia and nervus intermedius neuralgia may coexist; concomitant trigeminal neuralgia may be present.
3. Pharmacological treatment is similar to that for trigeminal neuralgia.
4. Neurosurgical intervention should be considered if first-line medication fails. Microvascular decompression (with or without sectioning of the ninth nerve and upper rootlets of tenth nerve) has high long-term success rates. Data on stereotactic radiosurgery are less favourable, and very limited for radiofrequency lesioning.

12.2 Glossopharyngeal neuralgia

See patient scenario in Table 12.1.

12.2.1 Clinical features

Glossopharyngeal neuralgia (GPN), also known as vago-glossopharyngeal neuralgia, is characterized by severe, brief unilateral stabbing pain, in the distribution

Table 12.1 Patient scenario

Features	Scenario
Sex, age	Female, 45 years
Location and radiation	Back of the mouth, pharynx, occasionally left ear
Characteristics	Occurs in paroxysms, both spontaneous and evoked
Severity and quality of pain	Intense, sharp
Provoking factors	Swallowing, coughing, speaking at length
Relieving factors	Nil. Over the counter analgesics no effect
Associated features	Nil
History of pain	Sudden onset 11 months ago. Lasted for 2 weeks. Following a remission of 3 months, pain re-started with its quality unchanged but with increase attack frequency
Effect of pain on life style	Office worker, off sick
Clinical examination	Nil

of the glossopharyngeal nerve and auricular and pharyngeal branches of the vagus nerve. This includes the ear, the base of the tongue, the tonsillar fossa, the pharynx, and the angle of the mandible. The attacks are typically triggered by swallowing, talking, yawning, or coughing. The frequency of pain attacks is variable and both exacerbations in the form of clusters of pain paroxysms and periods of remission tend to alternate. It is customary to distinguish otalgic and pharyngeal forms of the condition. A small percentage may develop pain-induced attacks of bradycardia, syncope, and very rarely asystole.

Diagnostic criteria (International Classification of Headache Disorders, third edition (ICHD-3) and International Classification of Orofacial Pain (ICOP-1), first edition)

A. Recurring paroxysmal attacks of unilateral pain in the distribution of the glossopharyngeal nerve and fulfilling criterion B.

B. Pain has all of the following characteristics:

1. Lasting from a few seconds to 2 minutes.
2. Severe intensity.
3. Electric shock-like, shooting, stabbing, or sharp in quality.
4. Precipitated by swallowing, coughing, talking, or yawning.

C. Not better accounted for by another ICHD-3 or ICOP-1 diagnosis.

12.2.2 Aetiology and pathophysiology

Vascular compression of the nerve root entry zones of the glossopharyngeal and vagus nerves is witnessed at operation in over 80% and is usually by a posterior or anterior cerebellar artery or vertebral artery. Similarly to TN, it leads to increased neural excitability and spontaneous firing. A local space-occupying lesion or a demyelinating multiple sclerosis plaque in the brainstem giving raise to GPN is exceedingly rare and more likely to cause glossopharyngeal neuropathy (see section 12.3.2). Mechanisms for syncope are related to ninth nerve connections with the carotid sinus. Rare familial cases have been described, hypothesized to be caused by mutations in a voltage-gated sodium channel gene.

12.2.3 Diagnosis and differential diagnosis

As with TN, GPN is a clinical diagnosis based on pain description and location. Clinical examination is usually unremarkable. While mild sensory deficits may be present in GPN, more extensive sensory deficits or a missing gag reflex should raise the suspicion of a glossopharyngeal neuropathy.

Conditions that may mimic GPN can usually be ruled out by history and clinical examination. Note, trigeminal neuralgia (TN) may coexist with GPN.

Differential diagnosis of GPN

- Other neuralgias:
  - o TN—confined to trigeminal distribution.
  - o Superior laryngeal neuralgia—can be triggered from cricoid cartilage, shoots to inside throat (see Chapter 13).
- Other neuropathic pains:
  - o Glossopharyngeal neuropathy—non-paroxysmal neuropathic pain (see next bullet point).
- Non-neuropathic pains—non-paroxysmal, continuous pain, pharyngeal pain provoked on swallowing, concomitant neck pain, generalized malaise may be present:
  - o Tonsillitis, pharyngitis, parapharyngeal abscess.
  - o Post-tonsillectomy pain.
  - o Retropharyngeal tendinitis.
  - o Eagle's syndrome (elongated styloid process).
  - o Tumours.

The patient in the scenario described in Table 12.1 was diagnosed with glossopharyngeal neuralgia (pharyngeal form).

12.2.4 Investigations

High-resolution three-dimensional magnetic resonance imaging (MRI) (fig. 12.2):

- Identification of neurovascular compression of glossopharyngeal nerve.

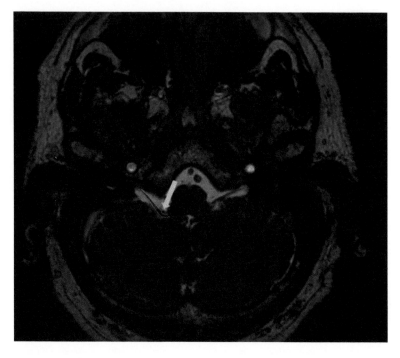

Figure 12.2 High-resolution three-dimensional magnetic resonance imaging of case scenario patient

Note compression of right glossopharyngeal nerve (marked by dotted lines) by posterior inferior cerebellar artery (white arrow)

- Estimate of severity of any compression.
- Exclusion of (rare) secondary forms of GPN (see section 12.2.2).

12.2.5 Treatment

All treatment is based on observational data only. Treatment is started using pharmacotherapy. If the patient fails to respond or develops serious adverse effects with first-line drugs, neurosurgical intervention should be considered as an early option.

Pharmacotherapy follows the same principles as treatment of TN.

Pharmacological management of GPN

- Carbamazepine and oxcarbazepine—first drugs of choice:
  (See Chapter 9 for details.)

- Other drugs to be considered in case of poor tolerability/lack of effect (if surgery not appropriate yet):
  o Phenytoin, gabapentin and pregabalin, topiramate, lamotrigine, baclofen (see Chapter 9).
  o No data on botulinum toxin.
- Application of local anaesthetic to the tonsil and pharyngeal wall:
  o Can prevent attacks for a few hours—not a long-term solution.
- Ultrasound-guided nerve blocks using local anaesthetic and steroid:
  o Mainly used in conjunction with oral medication. Additional pain relief lasting weeks. Suitable when short-term benefit is insufficient—as a bridging therapy before neurosurgery or in people with limited life expectancy.
  o Both intraoral and extraoral (peristyloid) approaches.
  o Avoid bilateral nerve blocks—risk for paralysis of the vocal cord.
  o Avoid blocks using neurolytic agents—major complication risk.
- Neurosurgical therapy.

The same rules of patient engagement as described before for other neurosurgical procedures apply. All data come from small case series, no head-to-head prospective or other controlled studies have been published. Table 12.2 summarizes studies published in the twenty-first century with a meaningfully long follow-up.

The patient in the scenario failed pharmacotherapy. MRI showed neurovascular compression likely involving the ninth cranial nerve. She underwent microvascular decompression (MVD) which was uneventful and has been in remission since.

12.3 Glossopharyngeal neuropathy

12.3.1 Clinical features

In glossopharyngeal neuropathy, the pain is continuous and described as burning, squeezing, or like pins and needles, with occasional superimposed paroxysms. There is usually a sensory deficit in the ipsilateral posterior part of the tongue and tonsillar fossa and a weak or missing gag reflex.

Diagnostic criteria (ICHD-3, ICOP-1)

A. Unilateral continuous or near-continuous pain in the distribution of the glossopharyngeal nerve and fulfilling criterion C.

B. A disorder known to be able to cause painful glossopharyngeal neuropathy has been diagnosed.

C. Evidence of causation demonstrated by both of the following:
   1. Pain is ipsilateral to the glossopharyngeal nerve affected by the disorder.
   2. Pain has developed after onset of the disorder, or led to its discovery.

D. Not better accounted for by another ICHD-3 or ICOP-1 diagnosis.

Table 12.2 Outcomes from selected surgical interventions in the twenty-first century

Procedure	No. studies No. patients	Immediate pain relief (range %)	Long-term pain relief (range %) BNI I–II*	Duration of follow-up, years	Mortality	Side effects	Comments
MVD	5 studies 211 patients	97% (91–100)	93% (90–100)	Mean 8.9 (range 1–21)	0	Hoarseness Dysphagia Facial paresis	
MVD + resection of IX and upper roots of X	4 studies 42 patients	93% (86–100)	95% (88–100)	Mean 5.5 (range 4–5)	0	Transient and permanent sensory or motor deficits	
Resection of IX with or without resection of upper roots of X	3 studies 115 patients	98% (92–100)	95% (92–100)	Mean 5.5 (range 0.5–17)	0	Transient and permanent sensory or motor deficits	Use when vessel not identified or difficult to move
RFL	2 studies 197 patients	81% (79–82)	54% (53–54)	5	0	Sensory changes	Target medial to styloid process Technically difficult
SRS	4 studies 41 patients	32% (0–82)	32% (32–36)	Mean 5 (range)	0	Delayed impact	Target where IX emerges from jugular foramen

BNI, Barrow Neurological Institute grades I–IV; MVD, microvascular decompression; TC, radiofrequency thermocoagulation; SRS, stereotactic radiosurgery.

12.3.2 Aetiology and pathophysiology

Tumours in the oropharynx, an elongated styloid process, ossification of the styloid ligament, Arnold–Chiari malformation, tonsillitis, peritonsillar abscess, trauma, vertebral artery dissection, and multiple sclerosis have been described as causes of glossopharyngeal neuropathy. The nerve may be damaged by direct trauma, compressed by a space-occupying mass or anatomical aberration, infiltrated by tumour tissue, or undergo inflammatory change. A multiple sclerosis plaque in the brainstem near the root entry zone may cause glossopharyngeal neuropathy.

12.3.3 Diagnosis, differential diagnosis, and investigations

Glossopharyngeal neuropathy is a clinical diagnosis, based on history (and clinical examination). Neuroimaging is mandatory, MRI preferable. Differential diagnoses include GPN and superior laryngeal neuralgia and non-neuropathic conditions listed previously.

12.3.4 Treatment

If the causative agent cannot be removed, the treatment will be symptomatic, based on pharmacotherapy and identical to that of trigeminal neuropathy (see Chapter 11). A pain caused by malignancy may be considered an indication for neuroablative treatment (radiofrequency thermocoagulation lesion, stereotactic radiosurgery) although experience with them is limited.

12.4 Nervus intermedius neuralgia

12.4.1 Clinical features

Nervus intermedius neuralgia is rare—there are less than 150 reported cases. It is characterized by brief paroxysms of pain felt deeply in the auditory canal, sometimes radiating to the parieto-occipital region. It is frequently associated with a constant pain experienced deep inside the ear that over time may become predominant. Patients may complain of altered lacrimation, salivation, or taste.

Diagnostic criteria (ICHD-3)

A. Paroxysmal attacks of unilateral pain in the distribution of nervus intermedius and fulfilling criterion B.

B. Pain has all of the following characteristics:
    1. Lasting from a few seconds to minutes.
    2. Severe in intensity.
    3. Shooting, stabbing, or sharp in quality.
    4. Precipitated by stimulation of a trigger area in the posterior wall of the auditory canal and/or periauricular region.

C. Not better accounted for by another ICHD-3 diagnosis.

12.4.2 Aetiology and pathophysiology

The pathophysiology of nervus intermedius neuralgia is complex and not well elucidated. Nervus intermedius neuralgia is part of Ramsay Hunt syndrome, although the virus usually causes a neuropathy. Neurovascular compression is generally thought to be the main cause, although is not uniformly present. During surgery, an artery (anterior inferior cerebellar artery or posterior cerebral artery) is seen covering the seventh/eight nerve complex, and it is not always clear if the intermedius nerve is compressed. Concomitant neurovascular conflict with the fifth and ninth nerves may be present. Multiple intrapontine connections between various cranial nerve nuclei make it difficult to make a judgement of the actual pain-generating mechanism.

12.4.3 Diagnosis and differential diagnosis

The diagnosis is based on pain description. No diagnostic tests are available. MRI rarely shows the miniscule intermedius nerve; a compression, if any, will have to be witnessed at operation.

Differential diagnosis includes nerves intermedius neuropathy, GPN, auriculotemporal neuralgia, and greater auricular neuralgia.

12.4.4 Treatment

Pharmacological treatment is identical with that for TN (see Chapter 9).

Surgery

Both MVD (fifth and ninth nerve), nerve resection, and their combination have been advocated. However, case series are small, retrospective, and patients with long enough follow-up are very few. One study reports a mean pain-free survival following nerve resection with or without MVD of over 6+ years.

12.5 Nervus intermedius neuropathy

Nervus intermedius neuropathy is characterized by unilateral continuous or near-continuous pain experienced deep in the ear. It is a very rare condition, the two commonest causes are herpes zoster infection and its aftermath, and prolonged neurovascular compression. Analgesic therapy is similar to that for trigeminal neuropathy (see Chapter 11).

12.6 Lay summary

The glossopharyngeal nerve alone, or in combination with the vagus nerve, is a rare source of neuralgia and neuropathy. Even rarer is nervus intermedius neuralgia (also known as geniculate neuralgia) and neuropathy. The diagnosis is based on patient history and is not easy as the quality of pain and the location are not always clear cut. Drug treatment is similar to that for TN and trigeminal neuropathy. Decompression surgery is favoured for glossopharyngeal neuralgia while nerve section is preserved for selected cases. Opinions on the best surgical approach for intermedius neuralgia are divided. Painful neuropathies are exclusively managed with medication, unless caused by malignant disease.

12.8 RECOMMENDED READING

Blumenfeld A, Nikolskaya G. Glossopharyngeal neuralgia. Curr Pain Headache Rep. 2013;17:343. doi: 10.1007/s11916-013-0343-x

Chen J, Sindou M. Vago-glossopharyngeal neuralgia. A literature review of neurosurgical experience. Acta Neurochir (Wien). 2015;157:311–21. doi: 10.1007/s00701-014-2302-7

Clifton SWE, Grewal S, Lundy L, et al. Clinical implications of nervus intermedius variants in patients with geniculate neuralgia: let anatomy be the guide. Clin Anat. 2020;33:1056–61. doi: 10.1002/ca.23536

Jani RH, Hughes MA, Ligus ZE, et al. MRI findings and outcomes in patients undergoing microvascular decompression for glossopharyngeal neuralgia. J Neuroimaging. 2018;28:477–82. doi: 10.1111/jon.12554

Kano H, Urgosik D, Liscak R, et al. Stereotactic radiosurgery for idiopathic glossopharyngeal neuralgia: an international multicenter study. J Neurosurg. 2016;125 Suppl 1:147–53. doi: 10.3171/2016.7.GKS161523

Singh PM, Dehran M, Mohan VK, et al. Analgesic efficacy and safety of medical therapy alone vs combined medical therapy and extraoral glossopharyngeal nerve block in glossopharyngeal neuralgia. Pain Med. 2013;14:93–102. doi: 10.1111/pme.12001

12.9 Continuing professional development

1. Severe neuralgic pain is reported in the throat. List the conditions that may cause it.
2. A patient complains of paroxysmal pain evoked by touching the left nasial fold, shooting toward the ipsilateral ear, and also severe sharp stabbing pain in the throat on swallowing. What is the primary diagnosis?
3. A patient with GPN is allergic to carbamazepine and oxcarbazepine. The treatment is commenced with pregabalin but there is no response. What should be the next action?
4. An elderly patient with several comorbidities has GPN poorly controlled with medication. An MRI scan shows an unequivocal neurovascular compression. MVD is ruled out because of operative risk. What do you recommend?

CHAPTER 13

Other cranial neuralgias

Francis O'Neill and Turo Nurmikko

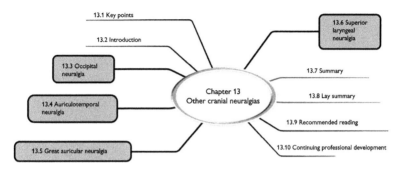

Figure 13.1 Plan of chapter

13.1 KEY POINTS

1. Lesser-known cranial neuralgias, including occipital neuralgia (ON), auriculotemporal neuralgia, great auricular neuralgia, and superior laryngeal neuralgia, are diagnosed on the basis of pain localization, pain provocation, and diagnostic nerve blocks.

2. In all of these, the commonest aetiology is thought to be nerve compression by an anatomical structure somewhere along the course of the nerve. Imaging should be considered in cases where clear-cut sensory abnormalities are present as secondary forms are seen occasionally.

3. The clinical characteristics of the neuralgias discussed in this chapter are summarized in Table 13.5.

4. Treatment options are based on observational studies only. Due to the dearth of published data, their effectiveness, especially long term, is not well established.

13.2 Introduction

It is not exceptional to encounter a patient who gives a classical description of painful paroxysms, but either the pain location or the triggering events seem to rule out trigeminal neuralgia or glossopharyngeal neuralgia. Such a patient may have occipital neuralgia (ON), auriculotemporal neuralgia, great auricular neuralgia, and superior laryngeal neuralgia. The nerves run a long course and may be subject to compression by muscles, fascia, arteries, bony abnormalities, or tumours at a number of potential sites, rendering them hyperexcitable and capable of spontaneous firing. The four conditions can be diagnosed clinically on the basis of their location, pain provocation, and diagnostic blocks. Definite sensory deficits within the nerve territory necessitate neuroimaging to establish the cause.

13.3 Occipital neuralgia

Table 13.1 describes a patient with ON.

13.3.1 Clinical features

ON is characterized by paroxysmal shooting or stabbing pain in the back of the head, often provoked by neck extension or rubbing of the scalp, and associated with subjective numbness. The greater occipital nerve (GON) is most often the pain's site of origin. A lateral occipital pain may be due to the involvement of the lesser occipital nerve (LON).

13.3.2 Diagnosis

Diagnostic criteria (ICHD-3)

A. Unilateral or bilateral pain in the distribution(s) of the greater, lesser and/or third occipital nerves and fulfilling criteria B–D.

B. Pain has at least two of the following three characteristics:
    1. Recurring in paroxysmal attacks lasting from a few seconds to minutes.
    2. Severe in intensity.
    3. Shooting, stabbing, or sharp in quality.

C. Pain is associated with both of the following:
    1. Dysaesthesia and/or allodynia apparent during innocuous stimulation of the scalp and/or hair.
    2. Either or both of the following:
        a. Tenderness over the affected nerve branches.
        b. Trigger points at the emergence of the GON or in the distribution of C2.

D. Pain is eased temporarily by local anaesthetic block of the affected nerve(s).

E. Not better accounted for by another ICHD-3 diagnosis.

Sharp pain or tingling evoked by gentle palpation of the nerve trunk of the GON, felt in the back of the head as high as up the vertex, is suggestive of ON. The

Table 13.1 Patient scenario I

Features	Scenario
Sex, age	Male, 49 years
Location and radiation	Back of the head, vertex, when intense radiates to forehead and back of the eyes
Characteristics	Dysaesthesia, with 2-second paroxysms superimposed
Severity and quality of pain	Moderate (visual analogue scale (VAS) 4–6), paroxysms moderate to severe (VAS 5–8)
Provoking factors	Gentle rubbing of scalp; pressure on nuchal line
Relieving factors	Nil
Associated features	Dizziness, tinnitus
History of pain	2 years of constant pain in the back of head, started several months after a whiplash injury, initially experienced on one side only before expansion to the other side
Effect of pain on lifestyle	Policeman, on sick leave. Stopped going to the gym
Clinical examination	Mild depression. Palpation of GON emergence at the base of skull results in pain shooting upwards toward the vertex. Reduced sensitivity to pinprick, bilaterally in GON territory (compared to vertex)
Diagnostic procedure	Two successive blocks by infiltration of the nuchal line with 2% lidocaine abolished scalp tenderness and provocation of pain for >45 minutes

diagnosis can be confirmed by two local anaesthetic nerve blocks resulting in temporary resolution of pain. For the GON they are performed at a point 1.5–2 cm below and 3.0 cm lateral to the external occipital protuberance, medial to the occipital artery, as shown in fig. 13.2 (note the more lateral blockade site for LON). Two common conditions that ON may be confused with are cervicogenic headache (arising from arthropathy of lateral atlantoaxial or C2/C3 facet joints) and myofascial neck and shoulder pain. If a diagnostic GON or LON block fails, diagnostic muscle trigger point injections and/or C2/C3 facet joint or atlantoaxial blocks (best left to experienced centres with adequate imaging facilities) are justifiable diagnostic procedures.

13.3.3 Treatment

Treatment is empirical as no randomized controlled trials have been published and no formal guidelines are available. Pharmacological management is similar

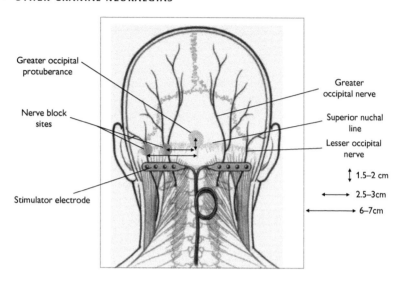

Figure 13.2 Landmarks for injection of occipital nerves and electrical stimulation

to that proposed for trigeminal neuralgia (see Chapter 9). For those with an unsatisfactory response, intracutaneous botulinum toxin injections as well as radiofrequency ablation of the offending nerve(s) have been advocated. Most refractory cases could be considered for decompressive neurosurgery or C2 ganglionectomy, although reported case series are very small and the true ratio of beneficial versus harmful effects are unknown. A less invasive intervention, occipital nerve stimulation, has been reported to provide meaningful long-term pain reduction in 70–85% of patients with refractory ON (fig. 13.2).

13.4 Auriculotemporal neuralgia

Table 13.2 describes a patient with auriculotemporal neuralgia.

13.4.1 Clinical features

Short-lived sharp, stabbing, or shooting paroxysms in the preauricular area, temple, and/or ear. It usually develops without any antecedent event.

13.4.2 Diagnosis

Characteristic pain can be provoked by pressing on the tragus or the periauricular region just in front of the tragus. Two local nerve blocks providing temporary pain relief will confirm the diagnosis. Important differential diagnoses include

Table 13.2 Patient scenario 2	
Features	Scenario
Sex, age	Female, 46 years
Location and radiation	Preauricular area, temple
Characteristics	Frequent paroxysms of 2–3 seconds' duration, and mild continuous background pain
Severity and quality of pain	Sharp, stabbing (VAS 4–7)
Provoking factors	Pressure on tragus
Relieving factors	None
Associated features	None
History of pain	9 months, developed without any antecedent event
Effect of pain on lifestyle	Reduced social contacts, no impact on her (part-time) job
Clinical examination	Normal mood. No sensory change, pain provoked by pressure on the tragus. No joint or masseter tenderness, mouth opening normal
Diagnostic procedure	Magnetic resonance imaging of the temporomandibular joint and surrounding tissue unremarkable. No diagnostic nerve block as would not be discriminatory. Moderate response to combined gabapentin and carbamazepine

temporomandibular disorder (see Chapter 15), great auricular neuralgia (see section 13.5), salivary duct and parotid gland-related pain (see Chapter 15), and referred pain from cervical structures (see Chapter 15).

13.4.3 Treatment

Recommendations for treatment come from few observational studies. Antineuralgic medications, such as carbamazepine and gabapentin, are reasonable options. There are reports of long-term effectiveness from a block of the auriculotemporal nerve lasting several months. Resistant cases may respond to surgical division of the lateral pterygoid muscle.

13.5 Great auricular neuralgia

Table 13.3 describes a patient with great auricular neuralgia.

Table 13.3 Patient scenario 3

Features	Scenario
Sex, age	Female, 36 years
Location and radiation	Before and behind left ear and upper lateral neck; occasionally deep in left ear
Characteristics	Paroxysmal
Severity and quality of pain	Attacks of sharp stabbing pain several times a day—episodes of spontaneous remission lasting for months
Provoking factors	Turning head to one side
Relieving factors	None
Associated features	None
History of pain	Started 3 years ago without any antecedent event
Effect of pain on lifestyle	No disability
Clinical examination	No sensory change, pain provoked by gentle tapping of the pain area, and maximum rotation of the head
Diagnostic procedure	Ultrasound-assisted blockade of great auricular neuralgia on dorsal aspect of sternocleidomastoid muscle abolished pain for several days

13.5.1 Clinical features

This neuralgia should be suspected when the patient presents with a history of moderate to severe paroxysmal pain around the ear provoked by turning the head to the opposite side. It presents as a remitting–relapsing condition, before eventually becoming chronic. At that stage, pain can be provoked by (1) touching the skin innervated by the great auricular nerve or (2) by compression over its course on the sternocleidomastoid muscle (fig. 13.3). Constant mild background pain is fairly common. The nerve supplies the skin over a large area from lower jaw to lateral neck (fig. 13.3). Neuralgia may follow head and neck surgery although most cases are idiopathic. Direct major injury to the nerve leads to continuous pain with sensory loss and is more appropriately diagnosed as great auricular neuropathy.

13.5.2 Diagnosis and treatment

The location of the paroxysms makes it easy to distinguish great auricular neuralgia from trigeminal neuralgia and other cranial neuralgias. In case of doubt,

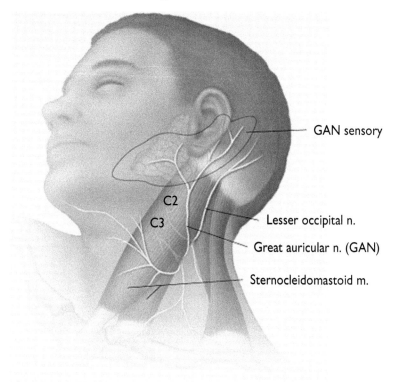

GAN sensory

C2
C3

Lesser occipital n.

Great auricular n. (GAN)

Sternocleidomastoid m.

Figure 13.3 Anatomy of the great auricular nerve

pain provocation by head turning readily confirms the same. Ultrasound-assisted blockade of the nerve as it travels along the sternocleidomastoid muscle is diagnostic and may provide long-term pain relief. Single successful cases have been reported from great auricular nerve stimulation.

13.6 Superior laryngeal neuralgia

Table 13.4 describes a patient with superior laryngeal neuralgia.

13.6.1 Clinical features

Patients describe a paroxysmal stabbing pain in the anterior neck, either localized or radiating to the pharynx or ear, and exacerbated by swallowing or coughing.

Table 13.4 Patient scenario 4

Features	Scenario
Sex, age	Male, 55 years
Location and radiation	Left lateral aspect of thyroid cartilage, radiating into throat, occasionally left ear
Characteristics	Paroxysmal
Severity and quality of pain	Sharp shooting, moderate to severe
Provoking factors	Coughing, swallowing
Relieving factors	None
Associated features	Hoarseness
History of pain	Started 6 months earlier after a prolonged respiratory illness
Effect of pain on lifestyle	Teacher, struggling at work
Clinical examination	No sensory change, stabbing pain provoked by compression of thyrohyoid membrane under the hyoid bone
Diagnostic procedure	Ultrasound-assisted injection of local anaesthetic into thyrohyoid space abolished pain temporarily

13.6.2 Diagnosis

Palpation of the lateral aspect of the thyroid cartilage that reproduces the pain is strongly suggestive of superior laryngeal neuralgia. Differential diagnoses include glossopharyngeal neuralgia, carotidynia, and Eagle's syndrome. Non-paroxysmal pain with local tenderness and no radiation from compression of the thyrohyoid membrane is usually due to local inflammation (hyoid bone syndrome).

13.6.3 Treatment

The thyrohyoid space can be identified using ultrasound and provides the site for diagnostic and therapeutic injections (fig. 13.4). The effect from a single injection is usually temporary but prolonged abolition of pain has been described following a series of blocks with or without steroids. Denervation of the nerve surgically and using Gamma Knife radiosurgery has been described but the long-term effectiveness of these measures remains unclear.

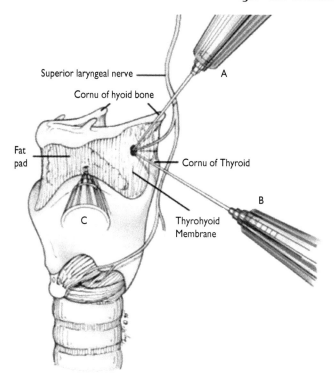

Figure 13.4 Position of the superior laryngeal nerve block

Reproduced from Preparation of the patient for awake intubation, Hagberg C. A., ed, Benumof and Hagberg's airway management 3e, Philadelphia 2013, Saunders p. 259 with permission from Elsevier.

13.7 Summary

Table 13.5 provides a summary of the key clinical features and the treatment options.

13.8 Lay summary

In this chapter, four lesser-known neuralgias are described. Pain in these conditions resembles that of trigeminal neuralgia but can be distinguished from it by location and provocation. Because of their rarity, little is known of the long-term effectiveness of nerve blocks that are commonly used. Surgery and nerve stimulation methods have shown promising results in more refractory cases.

Table 13.5 Clinical features and the treatment options

	Occipital neuralgia	Auriculotemporal neuralgia	Great auricular neuralgia	Superior laryngeal neuralgia
Origin of nerve	C2, C3	V3	C2, C3	Inferior ganglion of vagus nerve
Common compression site(s)	Trapezius aponeurosis, semispinalis capitis muscle	Lateral pterygoid muscle	Posterior border of sternocleidomastoid muscle	Thyrohyoid membrane
Precipitating event	Injury in many cases	None in most cases	None in most cases, may develop after any head and neck surgery	Infection or inflammation
Location of pain	Occiput	Temple, ear, preauricular, temporomandibular joint, parotid area	Lateral neck, ear	Anterolateral neck, radiating to angle of jaw
Pain paroxysms	Seconds, mostly less than 2 minutes	Seconds to 30 minutes	Seconds to minutes	Seconds
Pain provocation	Palpation over nerve in neck	Palpation over the nerve in temple, preauricular area	Turning head to one side, palpation over sternocleidomastoid muscle	Talking, swallowing, coughing, yawning Palpation over nerve in larynx
Concomitant continuous pain	Rarely	Frequently	Rarely	Rarely
Associated symptoms	Dizziness, tinnitus, frontal headache	Provocation of paroxysms by gustatory stimuli	None	Foreign body sensation/throat pain, hoarseness
Treatment options	Nerve block, nerve ablation, botulinum toxin, occipital nerve stimulation, surgery	Antineuralgic medication, nerve block	Antineuralgic medication, block	Antineuralgic medication, nerve block, nerve ablation

13.9 RECOMMENDED READING

Duvall JR, Garza I, Kissoon NR, et al. Great auricular neuralgia: case series. Headache. 2020;**60**:247–58. doi: 10.1111/head.13690

Finiels J, Batifol D. The treatment of occipital neuralgia: review of 111 cases. Neurochirurgie. 2016;**62**:233–40. doi: 10.1016/j.neuchi.2016.04.004

Keifer OP, Diaz A, Campbell M, et al. Occipital nerve stimulation for the treatment of refractory occipital neuralgia: a case series. World Neurosurg. 2017;**105**:599–604. doi: 10.1016/j.wneu.2017.06.064

Ruiz M, Porta-Etessam J, Garcia-Ptacek S, et al. Auriculotemporal neuralgia. Eight new cases report. Pain Med. 2016;**17**:1744–8. doi: 10.1093/pm/pnw016

Tamaki A, Thuener J, Weidenbecher M. Superior laryngeal neuralgia: case series and review of anterior neck pain syndromes. Ear Nose Throat J. 2019;**98**:500–3. doi: 10.1177/0145561318823373

13.10 Continuing professional development

1. List neuralgias presenting with pain in the ear (even if not the sole pain site)—include those presented in this chapter as differential diagnoses.
2. Which neuralgia classically is provoked by head movements?
3. Which neuralgia is suitable for neuromodulation treatment?

CHAPTER 14

Trigeminal autonomic cephalalgias

Cluster headache; Paroxysmal hemicrania; Hemicrania continua
Anish Bahra, Mohammed A. Amer, and Pravin Thomas

SUNHA (SUNCT/SUNA)
Matteo Fuccaro and Giorgio Lambru

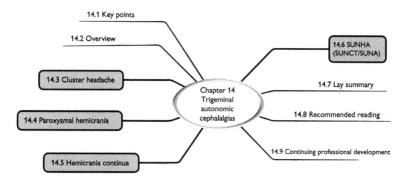

Figure 14.1 Plan of chapter

14.1 KEY POINTS

1. Trigeminal autonomic cephalalgias (TACs) are characterized by strictly unilateral head pain associated with prominent ipsilateral autonomic symptoms due to an increased parasympathetic output and sympathetic deficit. The clinical distinction is based upon the duration and frequency of attacks.

2. The pain in all TACs is best explained by a complex interplay between the peripheral trigeminal system, trigeminocervical complex in the spinal trigeminal nucleus, posterior hypothalamus, and upper cervical nerve roots.

3. Cluster headache (CH) is the most common TAC. In 80% of cases the presentation is episodic, where individuals have bouts of frequent attacks for several weeks or months, separated by prolonged remissions.

4. Other TACs may demonstrate an episodic pattern but are chronic or near-chronic in their presentation with short remission periods or none at all.

5. TACs are diagnosed clinically. Rarely, a TAC syndrome can be caused by secondary pathology. Brain imaging of new-onset cases is therefore advised.

6. TACs respond differently to various treatments. Subcutaneous sumatriptan is beneficial only for acute CH attacks. For preventive treatment, verapamil,

lithium, steroids, and galcanezumab show efficacy in CH; indomethacin for hemicrania continua and paroxysmal hemicrania; and lamotrigine, topiramate, and carbamazepine for short-lasting unilateral neuralgiform headache attacks (SUNHA).

7. Oral prednisolone, suboccipital steroid injections, and greater occipital nerve blockade are effective in episodic CH as a short-term interim treatment.

8. Patients with SUNHA who show neurovascular compression of the trigeminal nerve root on magnetic resonance imaging may respond positively to microvascular decompression.

9. For refractory CH, vagus nerve and occipital nerve stimulation have shown efficacy.

14.2 General overview of trigeminal autonomic cephalalgias

Trigeminal autonomic cephalalgias (TACs) are a group of primary headache disorders characterized by strictly unilateral head pain, usually within the ophthalmic division of the trigeminal nerve, associated with ipsilateral autonomic features.

TACs is an umbrella term for four separate headache disorders: cluster headache (CH), paroxysmal hemicrania (PH), hemicrania continua (HC), and short-lasting unilateral neuralgiform headache attacks with autonomic features (SUNHA). The latter is divided into two subtypes: short-lasting unilateral neuralgiform headache attacks with conjunctival injection and tearing (SUNCT) and short-lasting unilateral neuralgiform headache attacks with autonomic features (SUNA). In the International Classification of Headache Disorders, third edition (ICHD-3), all TACS except HC are categorized as either episodic or chronic. The former is defined by a period of 3 months or more between two attack periods (bouts) of 7–365 days' duration. These definitions are somewhat arbitrary but useful in optimizing therapy.

TCAs are rare and frequently misdiagnosed (see Chapter 4). The delay to the final diagnosis is several years.

14.2.1 Precision diagnosis of a TAC

The four TACs differ in attack duration and frequency, which form the basis of individual diagnoses and are at the core of the ICHD-3 criteria (mostly replicated in ICOP-1). It is worth remembering that these criteria are evolving and under constant review and should be applied with due clinical discretion. Patient presentations that resemble other TACs but fail on a single criterion are listed in the ICHD-3 under the heading of 'Probable TAC'.

Current classification demonstrates clearly that the intensity, quality, location of main or peak pain, referred pain, and behavioural response are features that TACs share to a variable extent (Table 14.1). The cardinal autonomic symptoms that include lacrimation, conjunctival injection, rhinorrhoea, and nasal congestion are similar in all four conditions. An often-underrated observation is that a minority of patients with CH, PH, and SUNHA describe low-level continuous pain between attacks. As will be discussed in later sections (14.3–14.6) of this chapter, some clinical features not included in the ICHD-3 criteria may assist the clinician in reaching the final diagnosis.

14.2.2 Pathophysiology

Our understanding of the pathophysiology of TCAs is still rudimentary. Converging evidence from neuroimaging, pharmacological and surgical interventions, and neurochemistry attributes much of the pain generation to excessive neural activity and the peripheral trigeminal system and trigeminal spinal nucleus, especially its caudal part with its multiple connections with upper cervical cord, hypothalamus, and higher cerebral centres and networks (see Chapter 3). This region, also referred to as the trigeminal cervical complex, drives the trigeminal parasympathetic reflex and causes most of the autonomic symptoms. Sweating abnormalities and Horner's syndrome, typically seen in CH, are thought to result from sympathetic dysfunction secondary to other events. Currently, individual TACs cannot be distinguished on pathophysiological grounds and substantially more detail is needed from research before it becomes possible.

14.2.3 Investigations

The majority of TACs are idiopathic with no clear aetiology. CHs have been rarely associated with intracranial pathology. In some guidelines, routine magnetic resonance imaging (MRI) with dedicated pituitary views is recommended as part of the assessment of a CH patient but such a practice is likely to yield mainly inactive pituitary microadenomas. Better justified is MRI of the brain in people symptomatic with TAC who are older at onset, and have atypical features or neurological abnormalities on examination. Pituitary-oriented MRI and pituitary function tests can be left for patients with obvious pituitary symptoms, or if a routine MRI is suggestive of a pituitary problem. Some patients with SUNCT/SUNA have been shown to harbour neurovascular compression of the trigeminal nerve root and may benefit from subsequent microvascular decompression. For a SUNCT/SUNA patient who is able and willing to undergo invasive neurosurgery, MRI applying the same imaging protocol as for trigeminal neuralgia (TN) should be considered.

14.2.4 Treatment

Therapeutic approaches must match with the diagnosis and vary considerably between different TACs. This applies to acute attacks and prophylactic treatment, and to both pharmacotherapy, surgical and neuromodulation treatments, and will be discussed in each section separately.

Table 14.1 Clinical features of TACS

	Cluster headache	Paroxysmal hemicrania	SUNCT and SUNA	Hemicrania continua	Side-locked migraine (subtype with autonomic symptoms)
Peak pain quality	Stabbing, piercing, pressing burning, throbbing	Stabbing, sharp, throbbing	Stabbing, sharp, burning	Throbbing, sharp, pressure-like, dull, burning, aching, stabbing	Throbbing pressure-like
Attack pain severity	Severe, excruciating	Severe to excruciating	Severe to excruciating	Background pain mild to moderate. Exacerbations severe to excruciating	Moderate to severe
Site of most intense pain	Periorbital, retro-orbital, temporal	Periorbital, retro-orbital, forehead, temporal	Eye, periorbital, retro-orbital, temporal, frontal	Orbital, frontal, temporal; less often occipital	Facial, temporal
Common sites of pain radiation	Occiput, neck, shoulder, teeth, jaw	Occiput, neck, shoulder, nose, ear, teeth	Nose, neck, vertex, occiput, teeth	Vertex, ear, occiput, shoulder, neck, teeth	Neck teeth
Attack frequency	1 every other day to 8/day, rarely more (typically 3–4/day)	1–40 a day (>5 per day for more than half the time) (typically 10/day)	1–200 per day (typically 60/day)	Continuous pain with exacerbations of variable duration	One to several times a week, less commonly daily

	15–180 minutes (typically ~100 minutes)	2–30 minutes (typically ~15 minutes)	1–600 seconds (typically ~1 minute)	Exacerbations lasting 30 minutes to 24 hours in one-half, 1–7 days in one-third, longer, or pain continuous, in the rest	4–72 hours, typically ~24 hours
Duration of attack (if untreated)					
Unilateral photo-/phonophobia	~50%	~50%	~50%	~50%	Rare (<15%)
Restlessness and/or agitation	70–90%	~80%	30–60%	~50%	Avoidance of movement
Circadian and circannual periodicity	Common (both patterns)	Rare	Rare	Rare	
Typical triggers	Alcohol frequently (50–80%), some solvents (VOCs)	Stress, relief of stress, alcohol, exercise neck movement commonly (20–30%), strong smells, weather, mechanical stimuli less commonly	Innocuous mechanical stimuli frequently (60–80%); exercise, light rarely	Stress, relief of stress, menstruation, alcohol	Stress, relief of stress, menstruation, missed meals, thundery weather, lack of sleep, too much sleep
Complete indomethacin effect	No	Yes	No	Yes	No

14.3 Cluster headache

See patient scenario 1 (Table 14.2).

Some 85–90% of CH patients have the episodic (ECH) and the rest the chronic form of the disease (CCH).

14.3.1 Clinical features

Diagnostic criteria for cluster headache (ICHD-3) (www.ichd-3.org):

A. At least five attacks fulfilling criteria B–D.
B. Attacks characterized by severe or very severe unilateral orbital, supraorbital, and/ or temporal pain lasting 15–180 minutes (when untreated); – during part (but less than half) of the time-course of CH, attacks may be less severe and/or of shorter or longer duration.

Table 14.2 Patient scenario 1

Features	Cluster headache
Sex, age	Male, 28 years
Location and radiation	Right always deep in eye, deep in the eye then radiates down the maxilla.
Characteristics of pain	Episodic, bouts on a regular basis from 6 months to 3 years, remission periods of 6 months to a year. Each attack tends to occur in the evening, most typically at 10 o'clock at night and lasts for about 90 minutes. Sometimes two attacks in the day
Severity and quality of pain	Severe (visual analogue scale (VAS) 10/10); pounding, shooting, stabbing, wrenching, burning, tingling, aching, tiring, blinding, unbearable, piercing, numb, torturing
Provoking factors	Aggravated by humidity, alcohol within 20 minutes of a drink can develop an attack of pain if in a pain bout period
Relieving factors	Nil
Associated features	During attacks: ipsilateral facial redness, tearing and eye redness, stuffiness or runny nose, sometimes a feeling of fullness in the ear, restless, can feel very hot, sometimes photophobia and phonophobia
History of pain	Started some 8 years ago
Effect of pain on lifestyle	Significant interference on activities of daily living when active
Clinical examination	Nil
Investigations	Normal brain imaging

C. Either or both of the following:

1. At least one of the following symptoms or signs ipsilateral to the headache:

   a. Conjunctival injection and/or lacrimation.

   b. Nasal congestion and/or rhinorrhoea.

   c. Eyelid oedema.

   d. Forehead and facial sweating.

   e. Forehead and facial flushing

   f. Sensation of fullness in the ear

   g. Miosis and/or ptosis.

2. A sense of restlessness or agitation.

D. Attacks have a frequency between one every other day and eight per day;
   – during part (but less than half) of the active time-course of CH, attacks may be less frequent.

E. Not better accounted for by another ICHD-3 diagnosis

Diagnostic criteria for ECH require the following:

A. Attacks fulfilling criteria for CH and occurring in bouts (cluster periods).

B. At least two cluster periods lasting from 7 days to 1 year (when untreated) and separated by pain-free remission periods of less than 3 months.

C. Typical bout duration is between 2 weeks and 3 months.

Diagnostic criteria for CCH require the following:

A. Attacks fulfilling criteria for CH.

B. Attacks occurring without a remission period, or with remissions lasting less than 3 months, for at least 1 year.

It is common for CH patients to report migraine-like symptoms during attacks, including nausea, photophobia (usually lateralized to the side of pain), and occasionally aura. Presence of profuse cranial autonomic symptoms, duration of attacks, and the patient's agitated behaviour during an attack distinguish CH from side-locked migraine (Table 14.1). More than other TACs, circadian rhythmicity is a common feature in CH. Cluster attacks can occur at set times during the bout, most typically waking the patient in the early hours of the morning or a couple of hours after falling asleep. A number of triggers (Table 14.1) will set off an attack during but not outside the bout.

14.3.2 Treatment

Management of CH is divided into *acute therapy*, used to abort an attack; *transitional therapy*, provided at the same time as prophylactic therapy is initiated; and *preventive therapy*, designed to prevent recurrent attacks for the duration of the bout (or perpetually in chronic CH). To date, no rigorously tested disease-modifying treatment has been approved. (The level of clinical trial quality and subsequent recommendation for any treatment shown is based on the criteria of the American Association of Neurologists.)

14.3.2.1 Pharmacological therapy

Real-world data confirms the effectiveness of triptans and oxygen therapy for acute therapy (Table 14.3). Arrangements for oxygen therapy require multiple steps, see Box 14.1. Intranasal lidocaine is administered with the patient holding their head in extension by 45 degrees, rotated towards the symptomatic side by 30–40 degrees, so as to reach the sphenopalatine ganglion. This treatment is an option for attacks lasting at least 45 minutes. Its effect is erratic. The main limitation is lack of an intranasal drug delivery device needed to overcome the common nasal congestion during the attack. Greater occipital nerve blocks (GONBs) as a single injection or suboccipital steroids as two injections 48–72 hours apart and oral prednisolone have shown efficacy in controlled studies and are suitable for both transitional therapy and prophylactic therapy for short episodes of CH (some weeks). Injection therapy may be repeated once or twice (regular injections lead to local skin and muscle atrophy).

The effect of verapamil in prevention of CH attacks may take up 2 weeks to appear. Verapamil tends to affect atrioventricular conduction by prolonging the PR interval. A pretreatment electrocardiogram is mandatory, and regular electrocardiograms following each dose increase is recommended and every 6 months once a stable dose level has been achieved. Lithium treatment can be used but is limited by an adverse event profile and the need for regular laboratory testing. Melatonin can be helpful in a minority but is generally well tolerated. Galcanezumab is a monoclonal antibody with an affinity to calcitonin gene-related peptide that was developed for the treatment of migraine. It is approved by the US Food and Drug Administration for use in ECH but not by European and UK regulatory authorities. It demonstrably has no effect on CCH.

14.3.3.2 Neuromodulation therapy

A significant percentage of patients with CH fail to achieve sufficient relief from medication, more so those with CCH. Non-invasive vagus nerve stimulation is effective in ECH patients as acute therapy but even if used this way only appears to reduce the frequency of attacks. Occipital nerve stimulation is effective in reducing attack frequency in CCH, an effect which remains stable for 5 years. See Table 14.4.

Two other invasive neuromodulations treatments have been advocated but their significance remains uncertain. Sphenopalatine ganglion stimulation

Table 14.3 Pharmacological treatments available for cluster headache and strength of evidence

Treatment	Mode of administration	Usual dose range	Titration	Main adverse effects	Evidence base/recommendation
Acute therapy					
Sumatriptan	Subcutaneous injection	6 mg; max. daily dose 12 mg	Minimum 2 hours between doses	Non-serious: vomiting, dizziness, fatigue, paraesthesia, tightness throat, neck	2 class I RCTs/established as effective in ECH, CCH
Sumatriptan	Intranasal	20 mg; max. daily dose 40 mg	Minimum 2 hours between doses	As above	1 class I RCTs/probably effective in ECH, CCH
Zolmitriptan	Intranasal	5 mg; max. daily dose 10 mg	Minimum 2 hours between doses	As above	2 class I RCTs/established as effective in ECH, CCH
Oxygen	Inhalation through non-breathing mask	12–15 L/minute	Up to 15 minutes	Well tolerated Caution in people with chronic obstructive pulmonary disease	2 class I RCTs/established as effective in ECH, CCH
Lidocaine 4% aqueous solution	Intranasal	2–3 drops	Repeat several times	None reported	1 class II RCT/possibly effective in ECH, CCH

(continued)

Table 14.3 Continued

Treatment	Mode of administration	Usual dose range	Titration	Main adverse effects	Evidence base/recommendation
Transitional therapy					
Prednisolone*	Oral	30–100 mg/day	Taper in 1–2 weeks		1 class I RCT/probably effective in ECH
Greater occipital nerve block**/ suboccipital steroids ***	Injection				2 class II RCTs and 3 class III studies/probably effective
Prophylactic therapy					
Verapamil	Oral	240–480 mg/day	Up to 960 mg/day	Non-serious: constipation, reduced blood pressure. Caution re: atrioventricular conduction effects (see text)	1 class II RCT, 1 class III RCT/possibly effective
Lithium	Oral	Variable, depending on compound	Up-titration to achieve a level of 0.4–1 mmol/L	Sedation, cognitive impairment, hypothyroidism, renal impairment	1 class II RCT; 1 class III RCT/possibly effective in ECH, CCH
Melatonin	Oral	10 mg	Nocte	None reported	1 class II RCT/possibly effective in ECH, CCH
Galcanezumab	Subcutaneous injection	300 mg	Once a month	Injection site tenderness and erythema	1 class I RCT/probably effective for ECH; probably not effective for CCH

RCT, randomized controlled trial.

Box 14.1 Oxygen therapy for cluster headache

Equipment
* Non-rebreathe mask (or demand valve mask).
* Two free-standing oxygen 100% containing cylinders (2000 L).
* Ambulatory cylinders (400 L).
* (Liquid oxygen (LOX) cylinder.)

Treatment
* 100% oxygen.
* Flow up to 12 L/min.
* Use up to 15 minutes at a time.

No response in 15 minutes, turn off oxygen. Use again next day at the earliest.

Different countries and regions have different oxygen delivery services and reimbursement practises. For an example of these, OUCH UK, a UK patient association, has produced an information leaflet. Go to: https://ouchuk.org/sites/default/files/downloads/o2_information_for_gps_and_neurologists.pdf

---

shortened CH attack duration in a pivotal sham-controlled trial but is not available for new patients. Deep brain stimulation targeting ventral tegmentum is reported to be beneficial in some CCH patients but adequately powered controlled trials are lacking and the method should still be considered experimental. It is in clinical use in few countries only.

A treatment pathway for CH is proposed here on the basis of efficacy in controlled trials and availability (fig. 14.2).

Several other neuromodulation techniques are being developed. A number of mini-ablative procedures have been reported to be beneficial but pivotal controlled trials are lacking.

14.4 Paroxysmal hemicrania

See patient scenario 2 (Table 14.5).

Chronic paroxysmal headache was introduced to the first edition of the ICHD in 1988 as a single entity. Over subsequent years, although the chronic phenotype remained the dominant sub-form, some patients experienced recurrent bouts

Table 14.4 Neuromodulation therapy available for CH

	Device	Application	Acute/ prophylactic therapy	Adverse effects	Evidence base/ recommendation
Non-invasive					
Vagus nerve stimulation	Non-invasive vagus nerve stimulation (GammaCore)	Cervical branch stimulation, 2 min ×3	Acute and prophylactic	Local erythema Transient dizziness	**Acute attack therapy** ECH: 2 class I RCTs/established as effective CCH: not effective **Prophylactic therapy** ECH, CCH: 2 class III studies/ possibly effective
Invasive					
Occipital nerve stimulation	Implanted occipital nerve stimulator	Personalized stimulation protocols	Prophylactic	Local post-surgical, no aftermath Hardware related (infection, implantable pulse generator dislocation, battery replacement)	1 class I RCT/probably effective as prophylactic therapy, CCH
Deep brain stimulation	Stimulator at ventral tegmentum	Personalized stimulation protocols	Prophylactic	Postsurgical, hardware issues	Several class III studies/possibly effective in CCH

RCT, randomized controlled trial.

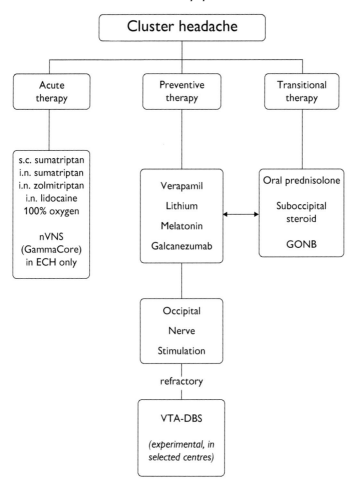

Figure 14.2 Treatment pathway for cluster headache

ECH, episodic cluster headache; GONB, greater occipital nerve block; i.n., intranasal; nVNS, non-invasive vagus nerve stimulation; s.c., subcutaneous; VTA-DBS, ventral tegmental area deep brain stimulation.

Table 14.5 Patient scenario 2

Patient	Paroxysmal hemicrania
Sex, age	Female, 41 years
Location and radiation	Always on the left side, trigger points preauricular mental region radiates to temple area and lower right quadrant intraorally
Characteristics of pain	Comes on suddenly, can last anything from a few hours to even 4 weeks. Mainly consists of continuous saw-tooth like pain but occasionally can be series of stabs that are very close together. Remission periods of few weeks, relapses last from a few days to 4 weeks
Severity and quality of pain	Severe (VAS 9/10) 'Knitting needle stabbed into face and then being turned'. MPQ: throbbing, drilling, sharp, heavy, exhausting, sickening, terrifying, unbearable, spreading, nauseating.
Provoking factors	Nil; aggravated by lying down, fatigue
Relieving factors	Indomethacin 25 mg three times a day; complete pain relief
Associated features	Increased salivation during attacks, restless
History of pain	2 years ago memorable onset of pain, given carbamazepine not effective, pulsed radiofrequency no effect, MRI shows no changes
Effect of pain on lifestyle	Significant impact on activities of daily living, no mood changes, difficult to work as a teacher
Clinical examination	Nil

separated by pain-free remission periods of months' duration. This led to the subdivision of PH into episodic and chronic forms.

14.4.1 Clinical features

Diagnostic criteria for paroxysmal hemicrania (ICHD-3) (www.ichd-3.org)

A. At least 20 attacks fulfilling criteria B–E:

B. Severe unilateral orbital, supraorbital, and/or temporal pain lasting 2–30 minutes.

C. Either or both the following

1. At least one of the following symptoms or signs, ipsilateral to the pain:
   a. Conjunctival injection and/or lacrimation.
   b. Nasal congestion and/or rhinorrhoea.
   c. Eyelid oedema.
   d. Forehead and facial sweating.
   e. Forehead and facial flushing.
   f. Sensation of fullness in the ear.
   g. Miosis and/or ptosis.

2. A sense of restlessness or agitation

D. Attacks have a frequency above five per day for more than half of the time.

E. Attacks are prevented absolutely by therapeutic doses of indomethacin.

F. Not better accounted for by another ICHD-3 diagnosis

Episodic paroxysmal hemicrania

Attacks of PH occurring in periods lasting from 7 days to 1 year, separated by pain-free periods lasting 3 months or more.

Chronic paroxysmal hemicrania

Attacks of PH occurring for more than 1 year without remission, or with remission periods lasting less than 1 month.

The distribution of pain is primarily within the ophthalmic division of the trigeminal but commonly radiates to C2 innervation territory, consistent with the physiological connections within the trigeminocervical complex (see Chapter 3). Rare cases of bilateral PH have been reported. Clinical manifestations of PH and other TACs are presented in Table 14.1. The high number of daily attacks (typically ten) should prompt consideration for a differential diagnosis of SUNCT/SUNA, from which it can be clinically distinguished by the duration of attacks and nature of triggers (when present). The ultimate diagnostic proof comes from the indomethacin test (see section 14.5.4).

There are anecdotal reports of intracranial pathology in patients with PH but the causal relationship remains unknown. It is not always possible in retrospect to temporally link a pathological process with the onset of the headaches, and its successful management by no means guarantees resolution of PH.

14.5 Hemicrania continua

See patient scenario 3 (Table 14.6).

The clinical features of HC and its response to indomethacin were first reported in 1981 by Medina and Diamond.

14.5.1 Clinical features

Diagnostic criteria for paroxysmal hemicrania (ICHD-3) (www.ichd-3.org)

A. Unilateral headache fulfilling criteria B–D:
B. Present for >3 months, with exacerbations of moderate or greater intensity.

C. Either or both of the following:
  1. At least one of the following symptoms or signs, ipsilateral to the headache:
    a. Conjunctival injection and/or lacrimation.
    b. Nasal congestion and/or rhinorrhoea.
    c. Eyelid oedema.
    d. Forehead and facial sweating.
    e. Forehead and facial flushing.
    f. Sensation of fullness in the ear.
    g. Miosis and/or ptosis.
  2. A sense of restlessness or agitation, or aggravation of the pain by movement.

D. Responds absolutely to therapeutic doses of indomethacin.
E. Not better accounted for by another ICHD-3 diagnosis
Hemicrania continua, remitting subtype
HC characterized by pain that is not continuous but is interrupted by remission periods of at least 1 day.
Hemicrania continua, unremitting subtype
HC characterized by continuous pain, without remission periods of at least 1 day, for at least 1 year

The pain is constant and unremitting, mild to moderate in severity, with superimposed more disabling exacerbations. The latter, in particular, can be associated with ipsilateral cranial autonomic features in 70–90% of cases. At least one migrainous features such as nausea, vomiting, and (lateralized) photophobia and phonophobia is present in 60% and one-half of exacerbations fulfil the criteria for migraine. The ICHD-3 does not recognize an episodic form but instead an 'remitting subtype' in which there is HC pain for at least a day.

HC has been associated with head trauma and intracranial surgery more frequently than other TACs, with identical presentation to primary HC. To date, any causality remains uncertain.

Table 14.6 Patient scenario 3

Patient	Hemicrania continua
Sex, age	Female, 48 years
Location and radiation	Left forehead, temple, and cheek consistently, radiating to upper neck
Characteristics of pain	Continuous fluctuating background pain, with daily exacerbations lasting from 30 minutes to 12 hours
Severity and quality of pain	Exacerbations: severe (VAS 9–10/10). Background pain VAS 2–5/10
Provoking factors	Relief of stress, exercise, alcohol
Relieving factors	Cold packs over pain area slightly helpful
Associated features	Lacrimation, eyelid swelling, nasal blockage. Restlessness during exacerbations
History of pain	6-year history of daily, near-daily episodes of headache. Occasional pain-free days
Effect of pain on lifestyle	Teacher, frequently on sick leave, eventually lost job
Past treatments	Trials with carbamazepine, pregabalin, amitriptyline negative
Clinical examination	No somatic findings. Mild depression
Investigations	MRI: no abnormalities
Treatment	Indomethacin 200 mg/day: complete pain relief. After 1 year developed catastrophic abdominal bleeding, requiring emergency surgery. Indomethacin discontinued. The patient ultimately obtained relief from a COX II inhibitor.

14.5.2 Differential diagnosis

See Table 14.1. HC may be difficult to distinguish from side-locked migraine, especially if it is associated with continuous interparoxysmal pain either spontaneously or with medication overuse. Liberal use of analgesic medication in HC may, in turn, augment the intensity of exacerbations making them mimic migraine attacks and induce medication overuse headache. Careful history taking focusing on the side lock, intensity of autonomic symptoms (note, not all HC patients have them), and profile of headache attacks with the help of pain diaries should assist considerably. Differential diagnosis with other TACs may be challenging especially involving patients who report continuous constant interparoxysmal background pain. Equally challenging are rare cases of HC comorbid with other primary headaches which is rarely reported (not surprisingly, given the presumably overlapping pathophysiologies). Judicious history taking, discontinuation of analgesic

> **Box 14.2** Is the pain responsive to indomethacin?
>
> Several approaches had been suggested for assessment of indomethacin in a patient with suspected PH or HC. Using a placebo control should be considered. The pattern of exacerbation (which may be erratic) needs to be assessed before the test (e.g. using a daily pain diary for 1 week).
>
> 1. Parenteral indomethacin (IndoTest*).
>
>   • 50–100 mg indomethacin intramuscularly. Only a complete or near-complete resolution of pain within 24 hours qualifies as a positive test.
>
>   NB: parenteral indomethacin for this purpose is not available in many countries.
>
> 2. Oral indomethacin.
>
>   • Starting dose 75 mg/day, increase weekly up to maximum 225mg/day:
>
>   • Week 1: 25 mg three times a day.
>   • Week 2: 50 mg three times a day.
>   • Week 3: 75 mg three times a day.
>
>   Stop at level at which complete resolution of pain is reached. If early response, consider administering placebo for 3 days. If not possible, test achieved effect by reducing dose to previously ineffective level (this will induce headache within 24–48 hours).
>
>   NB: use gastroprotection from outset.
>
> * Antonaci et al. Cephalalgia. 2003;23:193–6.

medication, and performing a subsequent indomethacin test is a powerful way to identify the conditions involved.

14.5.3 Treatment of paroxysmal hemicrania and hemicrania continua

There are no randomized controlled trials evaluating efficacies of treatments in either PH or HC. The relative rarity of these conditions undoubtedly is one reason. Anecdotal evidence suggests that triptans and oxygen are not effective as acute therapy for either condition. Treatment strategies in these conditions rely heavily on the use of indomethacin as prophylactic therapy. Testing for responsiveness to indomethacin (Box 14.2) serves both as an aid to diagnosis and initiation of treatment. Daily doses for control of pain are highly variable, ranging from 25 mg to 300 mg; the mean effective dose is 150 mg/day. Discontinuation or missed doses during active periods usually results in symptom recurrence within a day. Rarely, complete resolution of pain may take up to 2 months.

The most common side effects are gastrointestinal which can be improved with the use of a gastroprotective agent. Abdominal bleeding remains a risk and may necessitate discontinuation of the drug. Effect on the kidneys should be monitored. As with other headache disorders the drug does not alter the natural history. In one small case series, 15% of patients with PH were able to withdraw their indomethacin without headache recurrence. The goal is to maintain the minimal dose which provides symptomatic relief and tailor the dose according to activity of the disorder.

Some patients may not show a complete response to indomethacin. There is anecdotal evidence of effectiveness or other non-steroidal anti-inflammatories including COX-II inhibitors. No recommendation can be given to use of drugs effective in TN or neuropathy, peripheral nerve stimulation, nerve blocks, or drugs used for CH prophylaxis, because of sparse data.

14.6 SUNHA (SUNCT/SUNA)

See patient scenario 4 (Table 14.7).

14.6.1 Clinical features

SUNCT and SUNA likely represent the same clinical entity, with the latter associated with only one of the common cranial autonomic features which remains the only difference. They are distinguished from CH, PH, and HC on the basis of frequency of attacks and pattern of pain. Because of individual variability in these features so that they commonly overlap across all TACs, the importance of details of pain history and associated symptoms cannot be overstated. Both chronic and episodic forms exist. Together they are referred to as SUNHA and have very similar diagnostic criteria in the ICHD-3.

Diagnostic criteria for SUNHA, SUNCT, and SUNA (ICHD-3) (www.ichd-3.org)

Criteria for short-lasting unilateral neuralgiform headache attacks (SUNHA)
A. At least 20 attacks fulfilling criteria B–D:
B. Moderate or severe unilateral head pain, with orbital, supraorbital, temporal and/or other trigeminal distribution, lasting for 1–600 seconds and occurring as single stabs, series of stabs, or in a saw-tooth pattern.
C. At least one of the following cranial autonomic symptoms or signs, ipsilateral to the pain: 1. Conjunctival injection and/or lacrimation. 2. Nasal congestion and/or rhinorrhoea. 3. Eyelid oedema. 4. Forehead and facial sweating. 5. Forehead and facial flushing. 6. Sensation of fullness in the ear. 7. Miosis and/or ptosis.

D. Attacks have a frequency of at least one a day for more than half of the time when the disorder is active.

E. Not better accounted for by another ICHD-3 diagnosis.

Criteria for short-lasting unilateral neuralgiform headache attacks with conjunctival injection and tearing (SUNCT)

A. Attacks fulfilling criteria for short-lasting unilateral neuralgiform headache attacks and criterion B.

B. Both of the following, ipsilateral to the pain:
   1. Conjunctival injection.
   2. Lacrimation.

Criteria for short-lasting unilateral neuralgiform with cranial autonomic symptoms (SUNA)

A. Attacks fulfilling criteria for short-lasting unilateral neuralgiform headache attacks and criterion B.

B. Not more than one of the following, ipsilateral to the pain:
   1. Conjunctival injection.
   2. Lacrimation.

Criteria for episodic SUNHA

A. Attacks fulfilling criteria short-lasting unilateral neuralgiform headache attacks and occurring in bouts.

B. At least two bouts lasting from 7 days to 1 year (when untreated) and separated by pain-free remission periods of 3 months

Criteria for chronic SUNHA

A. Attacks fulfilling criteria for short-lasting unilateral neuralgiform headache attacks, and criterion B.

B. Occurring without a remission period, or with remissions lasting <3 months, for at least 1 year.

The ICHD-3 criteria are explicit and detailed and in typical cases allow for a straightforward diagnosis. Individual variations in pain descriptions make on occasion the differentiation between SUNHA and other TACs challenging. The key clinical features of SUNHA and how they compare with those of other TACs are listed in Table 14.1. One feature that makes SUNHA stand out is the presence of attacks triggered by cutaneous/intraoral innocuous stimuli applied ipsilaterally to the pain. Spontaneous and triggered attacks are reported by 56% of patients while 4% report only triggered attacks. This makes SUNHA the only facial pain condition together with TN in which the role of innocuous mechanical triggers is prominent, even if it is less than in TN where trigger-induced pain is a diagnostic criterion. The most common triggers, cold wind, light touch, chewing, and

Table 14.7 Patient scenario 4

Patient	SUNCT
Sex, age	Female, 42 years
Location and radiation	Right forehead, temple, and cheek, always same place
Characteristics of pain	Attacks of single/repetitive stabs, lasting 2–10 minutes. 5–10 attacks/day with mild interictal pain. No refractory period
Severity and quality of pain	Severe (VAS 8–9/10)
Provoking factors	Light touch, wind, brushing teeth/hair, chewing (also spontaneous attacks)
Relieving factors	Nil
Associated features	Ipsilateral lacrimation, mild ptosis, nasal congestions, rhinorrhoea. Restless during attacks
History of pain	3-year history of daily, near-daily episodes of headache. No remission period. No known precipitating factor
Effect of pain on lifestyle	Severe impact on work, social, and personal life
Past treatments	Initially diagnosed as TN. Failed to respond to carbamazepine and pregabalin
Clinical examination	Nil
Investigations	MRI: neurovascular contact with right trigeminal root, no morphological changes. Indomethacin test with max. dose of 225 mg/day: negative
Treatment	GONB with 30% reduction in attack frequency followed by lamotrigine titrated up to 200 mg twice a day, with 80% overall improvement of headache

brushing teeth/hair are similar to both conditions suggesting shared pathophysiological mechanisms behind provoked attacks.

There are differences that can be easily elicited from the history, the most obvious being pattern and frequency of pain attacks and presence of autonomic symptoms (Table 14.8). In SUNHA, unlike in TN, most patients (around 80–90%) do not experience any refractory period between attacks. Agitated behaviour that is reported in SUNHA is exceedingly rare in TN.

Table 14.8 Differentiating features of SUNHA vs trigeminal neuralgia

Feature	SUNHA	Trigeminal neuralgia
Predominant pain distribution	V1 > V2/V3	V2/V3 > V1
Severity of pain	Moderate–severe	Severe–very severe
Duration (seconds)	1–600	<1–120
Autonomic features	Prominent	None/sparse
Refractory period	Absent	Present
Preventive treatment of choice	Lamotrigine	Carbamazepine

14.6.2 Pathophysiology

While much of the physiopathology of SUNHA remains unclear, it is widely considered to involve peripheral and central mechanisms as in other TACs (see Chapter 3). It is possible that a contribution from the peripheral trigeminal is more pronounced in SUNHA. A prospective, large, cross-sectional within-patient MRI study demonstrated a trigeminal neurovascular conflict with the symptomatic trigeminal root much more commonly than asymptomatic root, and especially when compression induced-morphological changes in the root were assessed (80% vs 40%). Moreover, the topographical site of the neurovascular conflict tended to be superior and medial, known from TN studies to favour V1 presentation of symptoms. Findings were similar in both SUNCT and SUNA. Thus, some patients could benefit from microvascular decompression (see Chapter 10) but by the end of 2020 available data were too limited for firm recommendations.

14.6.3 Investigations

SUNHA is a clinical diagnosis based on detailed history and examination. MRI using a protocol optimized to show the posterior fossa as well as the relationship between the trigeminal nerve and surrounding blood vessels is the imaging method of choice (see section 14.1).

14.6.4 Treatment

Current evidence on SUNHA treatment is based on open-label case series. Both short-term (transitional) and long-term (preventive) management strategies are needed. Pharmacological therapy has a pivotal role in the management of the patient while invasive treatments are reserved for medically refractory patients (Table 14.9).

Sodium channels blockers are the treatments of choice. Lamotrigine, carbamazepine, oxcarbazepine, and topiramate have been shown to be effective,

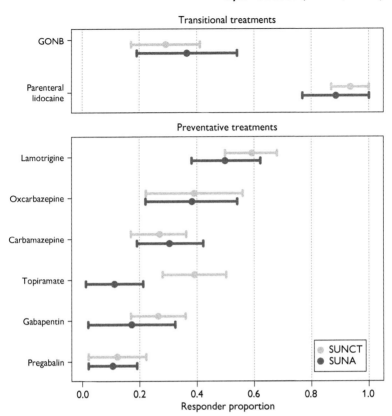

Figure 14.3 Effectiveness of common treatments for SUNHA (SUNCT and SUNA)

Pooled weighted responder proportions for treatments of SUNCT and SUNA, based on five published studies (N = 154). Responder = improvement of ≥50% in headache frequency/intensity/duration, or meaningful relief as judge by article authors. Error bars represent 95% CI bounds.

Source data from Lambru G, Stubberud A, Rantell K, Lagrata S, Tronvik E, Matharu MS. Medical treatment of SUNCT and SUNA: a prospective open-label study including single-arm meta-analysis. J Neurol Neurosurg Psychiatry. 2021 Mar;92(3):233–241. doi: 10.1136/jnnp-2020-323999.

both in episodic and chronic patients, even if higher dosages or combined therapy may sometimes be necessary. Lamotrigine has consistently shown superior effectiveness in various case series with one-half on average showing improvement of more than 50% and good tolerability (fig. 14.3). Other drugs used for neuropathic pain show lesser effectiveness, however, to a useful extent to be used in the clinic (fig. 14.4 and Table 14.9). Details of initial doses,

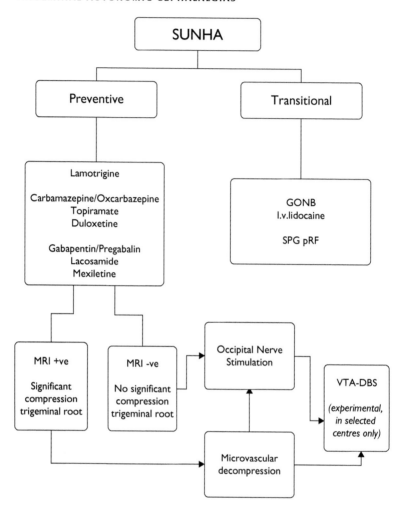

Figure 14.4 Treatment pathway for SUNHA

GONB, greater occipital nerve block; SPG, sphenopalatine ganglion; pRF, pulsed radiofrequency; VTA-DBS, ventral tegmental area deep brain stimulation

titration, tolerability, and side effects of these drugs can be found in Chapters 7 and 9.

Patients with severe bouts and those in whom invasive interventions are considered can be offered treatment transitional treatments, such as intravenous lidocaine, and greater occipital nerve blocks with local anaesthetic and steroid (GONB). In some centres, pulsed radiofrequency stimulation of the

Table 14.9 Recommended pharmacotherapy for SUNHA

Drug	Maximum dosage/day
First-line	
Lamotrigine	Up to 700 mg
Second-line	
Oxcarbazepine	Up to 2400 mg
Duloxetine	Up to 120 mg
Carbamazepine	Up to 1600 mg
Topiramate	Up to 800 mg
Third-line	
Gabapentin	Up to 4800 mg
Pregabalin	Up to 600 mg
Lacosamide	Up to 400 mg
Mexiletine	Up to 1200 mg

sphenopalatine ganglion has similarly afforded transient pain relief for some patients. Surgical treatments are by consensus considered for pharmacologically refractory patients.

From current evidence, which is at class III level, a *tentative* treatment clinical pathway may be recommended (fig. 14.4).

14.7 Lay summary

We describe here four severe nerve-related pain conditions of the head that appear similar. In all of them pain comes in attacks, is always on the same side of the head, and is associated with autonomic symptoms. The latter appear on the same side as the pain and include watering of the eye, swelling and redness of the eye and eyelid, flushing of the face, blockade and running of the nose, as well as sensation of fullness in the ear. Patients' descriptions of the pain details, however, are different for each condition and help distinguish them from each other. In one of them, SUNHA, sharp and brief pain is provoked by touch and this way resembles TN, and is helped by the same drugs. Another, CH, comes in attacks that resemble migraine but are shorter. Two other conditions, HC and PH respond to a single drug, indomethacin, exclusively and completely.

Regular medication that varies between the four conditions helps two-thirds of patients at least moderately. When pharmacotherapy fails, nerve stimulation methods can be quite helpful in stopping headache attacks or reducing their occurrence although this has been shown for CH only. An example of the first is vagus nerve stimulation in which a portable device is used by the patient to stimulate over the vagus nerve running in the neck (GammaCore). Another method is to stimulate the occipital nerves in the back of the head. This requires a surgical procedure in which the stimulator is placed under the skin to lie across the nerves (occipital nerve stimulation).

14.8 RECOMMENDED READING

Costa A, Antonaci F, Ramusino MC, et al. The neuropharmacology of cluster headache and other trigeminal autonomic cephalalgias. Curr Neuropharmacol. 2015;13:304–23. doi: 10.2174/1570159x13666150309233556

Lambru G, Rantell K, O'Connor E, et al. Trigeminal neurovascular contact in SUNCT and SUNA: a cross-sectional magnetic resonance study. Brain. 2020;143:3619–28. doi: 10.1093/brain/awaa331

Lambru G, Stubberud A, Rantell K, et al. Medical treatment of SUNCT and SUNA: a prospective open-label study including single-arm meta-analysis. J Neurol Neurosurg Psychiatry. 2021;92:233–41. doi:10.1136/jnnp-2020-323999

May A, Schwedt TJ, Magis D, et al. Cluster headache. Nat Rev Dis Primers. 2018;4:18006. doi: 10.1038/nrdp.2018.6

Obermann M, Nägel S, Ose C, et al. Safety and efficacy of prednisone versus placebo in short-term prevention of episodic cluster headache: a multicentre, double-blind, randomised controlled trial. Lancet Neurol. 2020;20:29–37. doi: 10.1016/S1474-4422(20)30363-X

Osman C, Bahra A. Paroxysmal hemicrania. Ann Indian Acad Neurol. 2018;21 Suppl 1:S16–22. doi: 10.4103/aian.AIAN_317_17

Prakash S, Patel P. Hemicrania continua: clinical review, diagnosis and management. J Pain Res. 2017;10:1493–509. doi: 10.2147/JPR.S128472

Wei DY, Jensen RH. Therapeutic approaches for the management of trigeminal autonomic cephalalgias. Neurotherapeutics. 2018;15:346–60. doi: 10.1007/s13311-018-0618-3

Wilbrink LA, de Coo IF, Doesborg PGG, et al. Safety and efficacy of occipital nerve stimulation for attack prevention in medically intractable chronic cluster headache (ICON): a randomised, double-blind, multicentre, phase 3, electrical dose-controlled trial. Lancet Neurol. 2021;20:515–25. doi: 10.1016/S1474-4422(21)00101-0

14.9 Continuing professional development

1. Name the two conditions that respond to indomethacin.
2. Which of the TACs is not associated with agitation or restlessness?
3. Have any of the available neuromodulation therapies shown efficacy for any of the TACS in controlled trials?
4. List three differences between SUNHA and TN.

CHAPTER 15

Other common non-neuropathic facial pain conditions

Pankaj Taneja and Lene Baad-Hansen

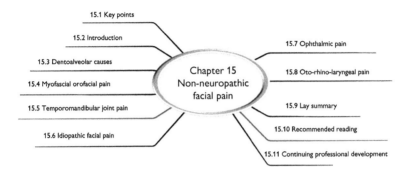

Figure 15.1 Plan of chapter

15.1 KEY POINTS

1. Non-neuropathic orofacial pain is common and mostly acute.
2. Most common is pain due to inflammatory conditions in the dentoalveolar complex.
3. Musculoskeletal pain affecting the masticatory system may become chronic.
4. Pain related to ophthalmic conditions is rare but it is essential to recognize and manage cranial arteritis promptly to prevent blindness.
5. Oto-rhino-laryngeal conditions are often acute.
6. Any of these can coexist with trigeminal neuralgia.

15.2 Introduction

Using the current classification systems, a short description of each diagnosis is provided. Uncommon conditions are not covered, and the reader is referred to the International Classification of Headache Disorders, third edition (ICHD-3), and the International Classification of Orofacial Pain (ICOP) for further information. See if you can classify the patient in Table 15.1.

Table 15.1 Patient scenario

Features	Scenario
Sex, age	Female, 65 years
Location and radiation	Poorly localized in upper right jaw region, radiates deeply through maxilla
Characteristics	Occurs in attacks, both spontaneous and evoked
Severity and quality of pain	Intense (visual analogue scale: 8–10 on 0–10 scale); shooting, gnawing
Provoking factors	Cold and warm food and drinks
Relieving factors	Analgesics, ibuprofen
Associated features	Nil
History of pain	Began 2 weeks ago, thought to be neurological, patient saw a neurologist; magnetic resonance imaging: nil noted. Carbamazepine on suspicion of trigeminal neuralgia: no effect. Referred for dental evaluation on suspicion of dental pathology
Effect of pain on lifestyle	Unemployed, married. Pain affects her social activities. Concerned about the cause of her pain, constant analgesics
Clinical dental examination	Carious lesion upper right first molar (16). Pain attack when air blown on tooth. Lasts 2–10 seconds
Investigations	Periapical radiograph of 16 confirmed deep carious lesion extending to the pulp of tooth 16
Diagnosis	Pulpal pain attributed to *irreversible pulpitis* due to caries extending to the pulp
Treatment and prognosis	Undertake dental treatment. Possible complications include periapical infection and may lead to the need of further treatment, e.g. revised endodontic treatment, oral surgery, or tooth extraction

15.3 Orofacial pain attributed to disorders of dentoalveolar and anatomically related structures

15.3.1 General

- Pain can be continuous, recurrent, or occasional and usually acute (<3 months).
- Evidence of a lesion by clinical, laboratory, imaging, and/or anamnestic evidence.
- In some cases, pain may refer/radiate to other ipsilateral orofacial locations.

15.3.2 Pulpal

- Characteristics of pain may include poorly localized, last a few seconds, and/or cause a sharp and deep sensation.
- Following a dental procedure, pain may occur hours to days after.
- Pain may occur from air, thermal, and/or sweet external stimuli, as well as occlusal forces.

15.3.3 Periodontal

- Patient may easily locate site of pain from biting or chewing.
- Swelling, redness, with/without pus formation.
- Characteristics of pain may include mild to severe pain, spontaneous, and lasting for hours.
- Following a dental procedure, pain may occur hours to days after.
- Tooth mobility/local deep periodontal pocketing.

15.3.4 Gingival

- Pain can be spontaneous. Gingiva may appear inflamed and ulceration can be present in some cases.
- Pain exacerbates when affected gingival tissue is manipulated.
- A source of trauma may be identifiable, such as ill-fitting dentures.

15.3.5 Oral mucosal

- Patient may report a burning, stinging, or sore sensation.
- Patient may report difficulty eating, speaking, and sleeping.
- Lesions such as ulcers, erosions, and vesicles may be present.

15.3.6 Salivary gland

- Pain may be experienced as acute or intermittent.
- Purulent discharge may be seen from salivary duct orifice.
- Redness of overlying skin of salivary gland can occur.
- Swelling of major salivary gland may be unilateral/bilateral.

15.3.7 Jaw bone pain

- Pain may arise hours to days after appearance of lesion known to be able to cause jaw bone pain.
- Bacterial, viral, or fungal infection may be present.
- Pain on palpation of lesion of jaw bone.

15.4 Myofascial orofacial pain (subtype of temporomandibular disorders)

15.4.1 Primary myofascial orofacial pain

* Pain is expressed as mild to moderate levels of deep aching or pressing pain in the masticatory muscles.
* Pain is modified by jaw function.
* Pain may occur episodically or unremittingly.
* Pain is often associated with impairment with regards to moving the lower jaw, chewing, and/or yawning.
* Pain may be referred to nearby structures.
* No cause of the pain can be identified.

15.4.2 Secondary myofascial orofacial pain

* Pain of similar quality and duration as primary myofascial orofacial pain.
* Pain may occur due to tendonitis, myositis, or muscle spasm.

15.5 Temporomandibular joint pain (subtype of temporomandibular disorders)

15.5.1 Primary temporomandibular joint pain

* Pain in and/or in front of the ear(s).
* Pain occurs in one or more episodes or unremitting.
* Pain may be provoked by either or both of:
  * Palpation of and/or around the lateral pole(s) of the mandibular condyle(s).
  * Maximum unassisted or assisted jaw opening, right or left lateral and/or protrusive movement(s).
* Pain is modified by jaw function.
* Pain may be referred to nearby structures.
* No cause of the pain can be identified.

15.5.2 Secondary temporomandibular joint pain

* Pain of similar quality and duration as primary temporomandibular joint pain.
* Pain may occur due to inflammation (due to, e.g. trauma, infection, crystal deposition, or autoimmune disorder), sensitization of the tissues, structural changes (such as osteoarthrosis, and disc displacement or subluxation), or injury.

15.6 Idiopathic orofacial pain

15.6.1 Burning mouth syndrome

- Patients report an intraoral burning or dysaesthetic sensation in the oral mucosa, recurring daily for more than 2 hours per day for more than 3 months (*NB: if <3 months, then probable burning mouth syndrome may be diagnosed*).
- No evidence of causative disorders or lesions are present.
- Negative and/or positive somatosensory changes may be reported.

15.6.2 Persistent idiopathic facial pain

- Persistent facial pain, with variable features, recurring daily for more than 2 hours per day for more than 3 months (*NB: if <3 months, then probable persistent idiopathic facial pain may be diagnosed*).
- Negative and/or positive somatosensory changes may be present.
- Pain may be described as either deep or superficial, and may radiate from face to mouth or vice versa.
- Pain may spread to a wider area of the craniocervical region.
- Variety of words are used to describe the character, and the pain can have exacerbations and be aggravated by stress.
- Clinical and radiographic examinations show there is no demonstrable local cause.

15.6.3 Persistent idiopathic dentoalveolar pain

- Persistent unilateral intraoral dentoalveolar pain, rarely occurring in multiple sites, with variable features, recurring daily for more than 2 hours per day for more than 3 months (*NB: if <3 months, then probable persistent idiopathic dentoalveolar pain may be diagnosed*).
- Negative and/or positive somatosensory changes may be present.

15.7 Ophthalmic pain

- Headache or facial pain may be attributed to disorders of the eyes (ICHD-3).
- Identify if pain is in or around the eye, if vision and/or visual acuity has changed, and if any signs of inflammation or trauma, such as subconjunctival haemorrhage.
- Ophthalmic causes could include occult trauma, posterior uveitis, optic neuritis, and chronic glaucoma.
- Non-ophthalmic causes should be considered, such as giant cell arteritis (fig. 15.2), intracranial aneurysms, and ischaemic attacks.
- Consult/refer to ophthalmologist if any doubt.

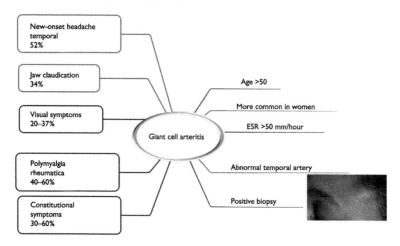

Figure 15.2 Giant cell arteritis
ESR, erythrocyte sedimentation rate.

15.8 Oto-rhino-laryngeal pain

- Headache or facial pain may be attributed to disorder of the ears, nose, sinuses, or other facial or cervical structures (ICHD-3).
- Pain can vary from severe to deep and boring, and from acute to chronic.
- Otic or nasal discharge may be indicative of the cause, for example, purulent from infection or cerebrospinal fluid from trauma.
- Hearing loss, itching, and tinnitus should be checked.
- Consult/refer to ear, nose, and throat doctor if any doubt.

15.9 Lay summary

Non-neuropathic pain in the orofacial region is likely a result of conditions involving teeth, jaw muscles, jaw joints, eyes, ears, nose, or throat. Knowledge of common non-neuropathic orofacial pain conditions will aid in defining the correct diagnoses and allow the clinician to establish the appropriate referral pathway for the correct treatment regimen. This chapter thus demonstrates the need for close collaboration between the medical and dental disciplines.

15.10 RECOMMENDED READING

See the classification references in Chapter 2.

Bird J, Biggs TC, Thomas M, et al. Adult acute rhinosinusitis. BMJ. 2013;10;346. doi.org/10.1136/bmj.f2687

Kuffova L, Forrester JV, Dick A. Assessing the painful, uninflamed eye in primary care. BMJ. 2015;4;351. doi: 10.1136/bmj.h3216

Sharav Y, Benoliel R, editors. Orofacial Pain and Headache, second edition. Chicago, IL: Quintessence Publishing; 2015. ISBN 9780867156805.

Siddiq NM, Samra MJ. Otalgia. BMJ. 2008;336:276–7. doi: 10.1136/bmj.39364.643275.47

15.11 Continuing professional development

1. What is the commonest cause of pain in the orofacial region?
2. Which orofacial pain is most likely to become chronic?
3. What are the commonest clinical symptoms for giant cell arteritis?
4. Name two orofacial pains that are classified as idiopathic.

CHAPTER 16

Role of psychological factors in the experience of trigeminal neuralgia

H. Clare Daniel

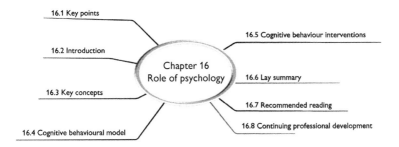

Figure 16.1 Plan of chapter

16.1 KEY POINTS

1. All pain, including trigeminal neuralgia, is the result of physical and psychological factors.
2. Results of investigations that come back as 'normal' do not mean that the patient is not experiencing pain or that the pain is psychological.
3. When working with people with trigeminal neuralgia, all clinicians, regardless of profession, must hold the cognitive behavioural model in mind. This will enable them to work more holistically and help in their interactions with patients.
4. Everyone experiences and responds to pain differently. There is no right or wrong response.
5. As part of a multidisciplinary approach, cognitive behavioural interventions can help people to reduce the psychological, physical, and social impact of trigeminal neuralgia on them and their lives.

16.2 Introduction

This chapter focuses on the experiences of trigeminal neuralgia (TN), but all content is relevant to other cranial neuralgias. This is because living with any persistent pain often has detrimental psychological, social, and behavioural consequences, which then influence the experience of pain and quality of life. The patient scenario is written by someone who experienced TN for 2 years prior to a successful microvascular decompression and yet the memories and distress remain (Table 16.1).

When a healthcare provider (HCP) is working with someone with TN, it is essential that they take a holistic biopsychosocial approach and have an understanding of how psychological, behavioural, and social factors are involved in what can be a complex scenario. Without this knowledge, the HCP will be taking a dualistic approach and neglect a significant proportion of the person's presentation. This will in turn affect their beliefs about the patient and decisions about interventions. This chapter is a guide to what any clinician needs to consider when working with someone with TN.

16.3 Key concepts

16.3.1 Understanding pain perception and experience

Clinical tip: everyone's pain is the result of physical and psychological factors.

Pain is an output, it is not an input. The often-used phrase 'pain receptors' is misleading because it implies that pain messages are transmitted to the brain. The ascending messages to the brain are not pain messages, they are electrical impulses initiated by chemical, thermal, or mechanical stimuli. They merely tell the brain about the body's external and internal environment. The brain is programmed to constantly assesses these impulses to detect changes and threats to which the person might need to respond. In essence, when the impulse reaches the brain, it travels to many regions spanning sensory, discriminatory, affective, emotional, cognitive, brainstem modulatory, motor, and decision-making circuits. Not all these areas are involved all of the time and the extent to which they are involved varies, which is why each experience of pain is different. The brain regions work together as a matrix to assess where in the body the impulse is coming from, what is the change that has been detected, and whether it is a threat. Only when the brain has made sense of the meaning of the impulses will it then produce an output. If the change is considered harmful, then the output is pain which alerts the person to remove themselves from the source of harm.

Pain is modulated by areas of the brain that are also involved in mood and cognitions; often called the 'affective brain'. Because different brain regions are involved in pain perception, the assessment of the impulses is influenced by genetic, cognitive, and emotional factors and memories. If someone feels anxious or low in mood, there is more activity in the sensory and affective regions of the brain and the stimulus is felt as more painful than if they were not anxious or low in mood. This is not the same as saying that pain is psychological; this is way that we all experience pain. Using the patient scenario as an example (Table 16.1),

Table 16.1 Patient scenario	
Features	Scenario
Sex, age	Male, 22 years
Development of pain	Classical TN managed with microvascular decompression and now pain free
Williams P (2015). *Life after Neurosurgery, Advances in Clinical Neuroscience and Rehabilitation.* Available at: https://www.acnr.co.uk/2015/11/life-after-neurosurgery/	I would sit at my desk, ready to revise, so grateful for being alive and pain free. But intrusive thoughts and images would invade my mind. What if it comes back? I suffered constant flashbacks of the worst situations I'd previously been in … like sobbing uncontrollably in public and getting odd looks or angry stares. Several times a week I would awake in a cold sweat imagining I'd felt pain in my face. I'd rub my lip viciously to confirm there was no pain … or was there? No, no, there was none, was there? Did I feel something just then? Had that been a tingle? If I drank cold water and dental sensitivity occurred, I would be inwardly petrified. I couldn't focus. I developed 'safety behaviours' like double tapping wood or my head in order to not 'tempt fate'. The anxiety and incessant head tapping often brought on headaches, and I'd get sudden panic attacks which would stop me in my tracks, whether I was walking in the street or in clinic, making me feel as though I was about to be violently unwell I felt ashamed. There were people who had gone through far worse than me—wars and assaults. And there I was, a twenty-year-old with absolutely nothing wrong with him, having these intrusive thoughts just because of a condition that most people had never heard of. I was a freak

because of his experiences of TN this man already feels anxious about the TN returning. Any change detected by the brain will be made sense of in the context of (1) images of 'the worst situations' such as sobbing uncontrollably, (2) memories of getting angry stares, (2) shame, and (4) anxiety. This increases the likelihood that pain will be experienced.

Recent research has used magnetic resonance imaging to determine whether changes in the affective brain of people with TN exist. Results are suggesting that their affective circuits are altered which may be associated with the comorbid depression and anxiety.

16.3.2 Pain and investigations

Clinical tip: the reported level of pain does not correlate with what is seen on investigations.

Despite evidence to the contrary, some HCPs believe that reported pain must correlate with changes/observations seen on investigations. If something is seen on the results of investigations then the pain is attributed to this finding. However, when the investigations come back as normal, some question the reality of the pain and might incorrectly label the pain as 'psychosomatic' or 'psychogenic' or the patient as 'malingering' or 'exaggerating'. This mislabelling has a negative impact on the HCP's perception of the patient, how they interact with the patient, and might influence the interventions given. As a result of this labelling, patients with TN are often distressed and angry about being disbelieved about their pain or being told it is psychological.

Believing that a person's pain is real and emphasizing to the patient that medical technology is not yet sophisticated enough to show the causes of all pain is the first step to ensuring a good relationship with the patient and appropriate treatment decisions.

16.3.3 Experience of healthcare

Clinical tip: patients' cycle of seeking a cause and cure for TN can be unhelpfully reinforced by well-meaning clinicians. This is why it is important to help patients understand their TN and why many interventions may not help.

Unfortunately, interactions with healthcare can contribute to the difficulties that people with TN experience. It can take a long time to receive a diagnosis of TN. A systematic review suggests that the mean onset between the first episode of TN and diagnosis is 10.8 months. People seek help from a general practitioner or dentist when TN is first experienced. However, some dentists and general practitioners know little about TN. This can result in misdiagnoses and/or a patient's ongoing search for a diagnosis and cure. During that search people might have unnecessary dental surgery and treatments and spend significant amounts of money on private consultations and/or complementary and alternative treatments. This cycle of seeking a cure is accompanied by enormous hope prior to appointments and then utter despair when treatments fail and the pain continues.

16.3.4 The relevance of the cognitive behavioural model

Clinical tip: hold an integrative cognitive behavioural (CB) model in mind when working with patients.

The CB model mirrors what is known about pain processing and perception and the involvement of both physical and psychological factors. The central tenet of the CB model is that our thoughts, emotions, behaviour, and somatic sensations

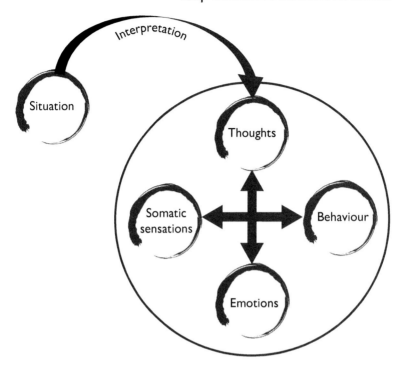

Figure 16.2 The cognitive behavioural model

are linked (fig. 16.2). If one changes, then one, two, or all of the others might change. This change will influence a further change in some or all of the others and so on. It is in constant flux.

16.4 Cognitive behaviour model

One important aspect of the CB model is that it is someone's *interpretation* of a situation that influences whether the cycle of thoughts, behaviours, and emotions are helpful or unhelpful. It is therefore people's thoughts about their pain and life with pain that can add another layer of difficulty to having TN. Holding the CB model in mind when working with patients will increase clinician's understanding of the patients' presentation.

16.4.1 Cognitions

> *Clinical tip*: understanding what patients think and believe about their pain and situation will help to understand their distress and behaviour.

In the context of the CB model, 'cognitions' encompass thoughts, beliefs, and mental imagery. The following examples could be related to the patient scenario but are the type of cognitions commonly verbalized by people with TN. As the CB model suggests, these cognitions will lead to an increase in distress.

- *Thoughts:*
  - 'I should be grateful that I'm now pain free, but I'm just so scared it'll return.'
  - 'I can't concentrate on my revision. I'm going to fail my degree, I won't get a good job and I won't be able to afford rent. I'll have nowhere to live.'
- *Beliefs:*
  - 'My TN is caused by cancer, but no one can find it. I might die. I'm scared.'
- *Mental imagery:*
  - 'I see it as a creeping faceless being that's lurking in the dark corners. I know it's going to attack but I don't know when.'

As the patient scenario highlights, it is not just during a TN attack that thoughts are distressing. Even during the pain-free periods or after a successful medical intervention people can be plagued by memories and thoughts of their TN. It is the unpredictability of the pain that results in 'What if ...?' thoughts; 'What if I go outside in the wind and it triggers an attack?'; 'What if I shave and it triggers an attack?'; 'What if I meet friends and have an attack when we're eating dinner?' Knowing the answers to these 'What if ...?' questions can help to understand the fears of people with TN. These fears tend to be about being out of the home and not being able to return; other people's perception of them during an attack (patient scenario: 'getting odd looks or angry stares'); feeling ashamed (patient scenario: 'people who had gone through far worse than me').

16.4.2 Emotions

Clinical tip: we cannot make a judgement about whether someone's level distress is too low or too high.

When we feel anxious, it is often associated with a perception of being under threat; when we feel depressed, it is often due to experiencing losses; when we feel angry, it is because we perceive something as unfair; when we feel frustrated, it is because something is getting in our way.

- TN pain is threatening and so people feel anxious.
- TN can result in losses (e.g. loss of a job because they are unable to concentrate; loss of friends because they find talking for a long time difficult) and so people experience low mood or clinical depression.
- Having TN can feel so unfair and so people can feel angry.
- TN can be an enormous obstacle that gets in the way of achieving even day-to-day activities and so people can feel frustrated.

Some people with TN report symptoms that are akin to those of post-traumatic stress disorder and while they might not reach the diagnostic criteria for post-traumatic stress disorder, they do suffer in similar ways (Jiang, 2019). As in the patient scenario, they experience intrusive symptoms such as flashbacks and nightmares, avoid reminders of TN, and experience alterations in mood and increased arousal.

16.4.3 Behaviours

Clinical tip: even what appear to be the oddest of behaviours make sense when we understand the thoughts and beliefs that drive them.

Our cognitions and emotions influence our behaviour. When our thoughts are about a perceived physical or psychological threat, we become fearful and we engage in behaviours that we believe will protect us. These behaviours can be called 'safety behaviours' (see Table 16.1) and refer to overt or covert behaviours that we think will prevent a feared event from occurring. People with TN carry out safety behaviours because they believe it will prevent an attack of TN. For example, they might:

- Wear a woolly scarf *every* time they go outside.
- Always make sure food is very soft.
- Stop shaving.
- Engage in subtle behaviours such as the tapping described in the patient scenario (Table 16.1).

Initially, these safety behaviours provide a sense of safety. However, there are significant disadvantages to them:

- They prevent disconfirmation of the belief that an attack *will* happen, so the absence of a TN attack is attributed to the safety behaviour. Therefore, beliefs such as 'I didn't get an attack because I was wearing a scarf' persist, as does the safety behaviour.
- Safety behaviours can lead to other, more limiting behaviours. For example, wearing a scarf is appropriate in cold weather but this can generalize to warmer weather and can cause difficulties such as feeling uncomfortably hot or attracting jibes from friends. Someone's response to these might be a more limiting behaviour, for example, stopping going out which can lead to isolation and low mood.

Vicious cycles and reduced quality of life

It is easy to see how vicious cycles of unhelpful thoughts, emotions and behaviours begin until eventually life is consumed by TN, fear, low mood, avoidance behaviours, and isolation (fig. 16.3).

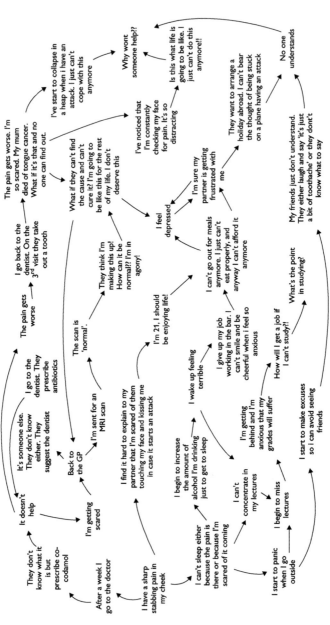

Figure 16.3 Example of the vicious cycles and secondary effects of living with TN

16.5 Cognitive behavioural interventions

There is a plethora of high-quality research on the psychological, physical, and social impact of persistent pain and on CB interventions to reduce this impact. However this has been slow to filter into the TN research and clinical field although there are signs that this might be changing.

CB interventions do not aim to change the TN, but to change people's relationship with the TN. They aim to help people:

- Understand TN and subsequently be less fearful of it.
- Recognize their own vicious cycles and develop cognitive and behavioural strategies to break these cycles.
- Develop cognitive and behavioural strategies to use during and after an attack.
- Develop strategies to begin to return to activities that they fear but would like to do (e.g. eating in public, walking in the wind, tolerating touch).

A recent study suggested that CB interventions in a group format help people to reduce the impact of TN. Many healthcare services do not have the resources or patient numbers to run these groups; however, a referral to a psychologist and a physiotherapist who have an understanding of TN could help the patient.

16.5.1 Non-psychological healthcare providers and cognitive behavioural principles

Healthcare providers without any psychological training have an important role when working with people with TN. In addition to the clinical tips in this chapter the following are important:

1. Discover what the patient believes is causing their pain by simply saying 'It really helps me when I know what people think is causing their TN, what do you think is causing yours?' HCPs can explain the reason for TN but if the patient believes it is caused by, for example, cancer or multiple sclerosis when it is not, then this belief needs to be voiced for the HCP to help change it and prevent the patient from returning home with a lingering doubt and fear that can grow.

2. All patients are individuals; listen to what each patient is telling us and without judgement. It might sound strange to say listen to the patient given that this is what HCPs do on a daily basis. However, HCPs are not as good at listening as they might think. The main reason for patients' formal complaints in healthcare settings is poor communication. Patients want to be listened to, given clear information about their care, and treated with respect. Many of us believe that we are listening but we are actually thinking about what to say next. We might also place our

own value system and experiences onto what the patient is saying and add a layer of unhelpful judgement.

3. Normalize people's experience of TN without giving the impression that we are saying 'Don't worry, this is normal' because this will undermine their experiences. Many people with the condition have not met anyone else with TN. Telling them that 'What you're telling me is what many other people with TN say. It is a difficult condition to live with' might re-assure people that their experiences and responses to TN are normal.

4. Be mindful of the words we use; what we think is a benign word or phrase could cause concern and distress for patients. They will interpret what we say in the context of their own experiences, memories, and mood and so the meaning of what we are saying might be changed.

   • For example, TN is called the 'suicide disease' probably to acknowledge how difficult it can be to live with TN. However, if a patient comes to clinic already fearful and they are told that TN is called the suicide disease, this will probably increase their distress and hopelessness and have a significant detrimental effect on their mood which might feed into the previously discussed vicious cycles.

   • 'Maybe you can distract yourself by doing something you enjoy' is a common suggestion to people with TN. Many people with TN feel frustrated when they hear this. During a TN attack people cannot distract themselves—the pain is all consuming. Suggesting distraction gives people the message that we do not understand their experiences. Even the suggestion of distracting themselves between attacks can be met with frustration. We can give the same message without saying 'distraction'. For example, 'I'm wondering if there is something enjoyable that you used to do but you have stopped and maybe you could start again slowly?'

   • Avoid saying 'I understand', because we never fully understand what anyone is experiencing. 'I understand' is often met with frustration or anger. Instead say something such as 'It sounds very difficult for you'. That might be met with 'Of course it's very difficult!' but we have acknowledged their difficulty and some patients appreciate this and feel understood.

16.6 Lay summary

TN is an unpredictable and distressing pain that can have psychological, behav-ioural, and social consequences on people and their lives. It is important that all clinicians working with people with TN have an understanding of the role of psychological factors in pain processing and perception to enable them to make sense of the person's presentation and to work with them within a holistic framework. The CB model highlights the interaction between people's TN, their thoughts, emotions, and behaviour. If all clinicians hold the model in their mind, it will help them to understand the difficulties that people experience and help with their relationship with patients. There is some evidence that a multidisciplinary approach to TN, including CB interventions, can help people who are suffering with TN.

16.7 RECOMMENDED READING

Castro AR, Siqueira SR, Perissinotti DM, et al. Emotional aspects of chronic orofacial pain and surgical treatment. Int J Surg. 2009;7:196–9. doi: 10.1016/j.ijsu.2009.02.002

Daniel HC, Poole JJ, Klein H, et al. Cognitive behavioural therapy for patients with trigeminal neuralgia: a feasibility study. J Oral Facial Pain Headache. 2021;**35**:30–4. doi: 10.11607/ofph.2664

David L. Using CBT in General Practice: The 10 Minute CBT Handbook, second edition. Banbury: Scion Publishing Ltd; 2013.

Fullen BM, Blake C, Horan S, et al. Ulysses: the effectiveness of a multidisciplinary cognitive behavioural pain management programme—an 8-year review. Ir J Med Sci. 2014;**183**:265–75. doi: 10.1007/s11845-013-1002-2

Melek LN, Devine M, Renton T. The psychosocial impact of orofacial pain in trigeminal neuralgia patients: a systematic review. Int J Oral Maxfac Surg. 2018;**47**:869–78. doi: 10.1016/j.ijom.2018.02.006.

Websites

British Pain Society: a website for healthcare providers and people with pain. https://www.britishpainsociety.org/people-with-pain/

HealthTalk.org: a website to help people understand long-term conditions. https://healthtalk.org/chronic-pain/overview

Live well with pain: a website for healthcare providers focusing on understanding persistent pain, talking to people with pain, and supporting them to manage their pain; also for patients. https://livewellwithpain.co.uk

16.8 Continuing professional development

1. List four psychosocial impacts of TN and other cranial neuralgias.
2. What are the four elements of the CB model?
3. Which of the following are helpful statements to say to patients?
   a. What do you think is causing your TN?
   b. Don't worry, this is normal.
   c. It sounds very difficult for you.
   d. I understand what you are experiencing.

CHAPTER 17

Patient support groups

Jillie Abbott, Claire Patterson, and Elena Semino

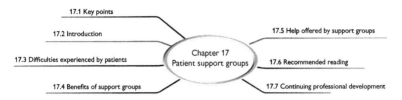

Figure 17.1 Plan of chapter

17.1 KEY POINTS

1. Patient support groups provide mutual support to patients and help to validate their experiences.
2. Patients face considerable difficulties and obstacles, beginning with getting a correct diagnosis through to getting the correct treatments by the right professionals at the right time.
3. Medical advisory boards form part of support groups and provide guidance-based, high-quality research evidence.
4. Misinformation is common on the internet and support groups try to ensure that their information is accurate and reliable.
5. Being listened to by fellow sufferers can help to reduce fear, isolation, anxiety, and depression.
6. Help from support groups is offered through a range of methods including telephone, email, leaflets, internet and conferences.
7. Members of support groups provide input into the design of research studies and can help in the recruitment of patients into clinical trials.
8. Support groups working with larger organizations can help to influence policies and increase awareness of trigeminal neuralgia among healthcare professionals.

17.2 Introduction

> There isn't one person with trigeminal neuralgia I know whose life has not been altered by the experience.
>
> Claire Patterson

> My life has changed beyond all recognition as a result of having TN. I
> was forced to sell my business, my marriage broke up and I lost many
> friends because, in effect, I was self-isolating. Covid 19 isolation is a
> doddle for me, I've been there before and I'm still wearing the T-shirt.
>
> Jillie Abbott

Trigeminal neuralgia (TN) really is life changing, in so many ways. The fear factor
and the feeling of isolation cannot be overstated. Likewise, the value of a strong
support group cannot be overstressed. Dr Peter Jannetta, pioneer of the microvascular decompression procedure, spoke at the first Trigeminal Neuralgia
Association Conference in the USA in 1990, which was only open to support
group leaders. The title of his talk was 'The Difference You Have Made!' His
recognition of support group leaders and their efforts speaks volumes. He understood their value and the support and guidance they can give. He composed and
sang the song shown in fig. 17.2 at one of the USA conferences.

In this chapter, we introduce the different types of help that are provided by
support groups. In the English-speaking world, there are national groups: the
Facial Pain Association USA, Trigeminal Neuralgia Association UK (TNA UK),
Trigeminal Neuralgia Association Australia, and Trigeminal Neuralgia Association
Canada, and there are also groups in Denmark and Italy. In the UK, there is a
patient support group called OUCH UK for patients with trigeminal autonomic
cephalalgias.

17.3 Difficulties experienced by patients

Over the years, the support groups have identified some of the key issues that
face people with TN. These are summarized in fig. 17.3.

17.3.1 Getting the correct diagnosis

As TN is rare, it can take a long time to get a diagnosis, especially if patients do
not appear 'to fit' the recognized criteria, for example, 'too young to have TN.'

17.3.2 Impact of severe pain

TN is invisible and unpredictable and both healthcare professionals (HCPs) and
the public fail to recognize the severity of the pain and its impact on quality of life:

> To have pain and be questioned about the reality of the pain is extremely difficult
> to handle and depressing. When a person is believed about their pain, they will
> be treated with the same respect and dignity as anyone else. (Penney Cowan,
> Founder and CEO, the American Chronic Pain Association)

TIC DOULOUREUX MY DARLING

Got my face pain, out of the blue
Got my face pain, out of the blue
Got my face pain, out of the blue
What did I do my Darling.

Saw a dentist as did you
Saw a dentist as did you
Saw a dentist as did you
He took my teeth out Darling.

Saw my doctor as did you
Saw my doctor as did you
Saw my doctor as did you
He didn't help my Darling.

Saw a neurologist as did you
He diagnosed it that is true
He diagnosed it that is true
Tic douloureux, my Darling.
Tegretol, Dilantin, Baclofen
Dilantin, Baclofen, Tegretol
Baclofen, Dilantin, Tegretol
Slept all the time my, Darling.

Operation is for you
Operation is for you
Operation is for you
Said Dr. so & so, my Darling.

All the surgeons do what they do
Help most of us, hurt a few
Help most of us, maybe you
Tic Douloureux, my Darling.

Tic doulo, tic doulo, tic douloureux
Tic doulo, tic doulo, tic douloureux
Tic doulo, tic doulo, tic douloureux
Tic Douloureux, my Darling.

Figure 17.2 Song written and sung by Dr Peter Jannetta at a USA Support Group meeting
Sung to the tune of Waltzing Matilda, signed by Peter Jannetta.

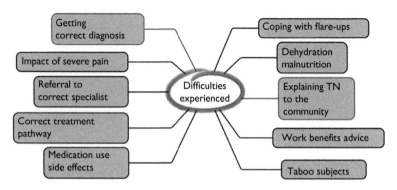

Figure 17.3 Difficulties encountered by patients with TN from the patients' perspective

17.3.3 Referral to the correct specialist

Since most of the early symptoms of TN are felt in the teeth and jaw, the dentist is usually the first clinician seen by the patient. But all too often, the dentist will pursue a course of root canal work, splints, and extractions. Sometimes the dentist refers the patient to a maxillofacial surgeon rather than a neurologist or pain specialist.

17.3.4 Correct treatment pathway

Many doctors continue to treat their patients long after surgical options should have been discussed. Rather than wait too long, it is important that patients see a neurosurgeon who can offer a range of treatments.

17.3.5 Medication use and side effects

- Some patients will take antiepileptic drugs like painkillers because they have not been told otherwise. The medications are then ineffective, so patients lose faith.
- Patients lack instruction on how to take medication—'slowly up and slowly down', before meals if necessary.
- Many fail to be told to keep in touch with their HCP if their drug level is not effective.
- As dosages increase, so may side effects—'feeling like a zombie', 'brain fog', and 'being spaced out' are common complaints but patients are often not warned about these.
- Knowing others suffer side effects such as sleepiness, nausea, confusion, and disorientation is comforting; many are not told that a rash can be dangerous.

- It is not made clear that, given time and perseverance, the right balance to maintain reasonable pain control and fewer side effects can usually be achieved.

17.3.6 Coping with flare-ups

It can be very difficult to get help and significant others often feel helpless as they do not know where to turn. Patients need to have 'flare-up plans'. Long-term sufferers will have amassed a myriad of tips and suggestions for those struggling to cope with an intense pain flare-up. Some of these are shown in Box 17.1.

17.3.7 Dehydration and malnutrition

Some patients fare so badly that they become undernourished, even sometimes dehydrated because drinking is impossible and admission to hospital may then be necessary.

17.3.8 Explaining TN to the community

Sufferers may struggle because even their loved ones fail to understand the intensity and the unpredictability of the pain. Colleagues or employers may consider they are 'swinging the lead' because there is no visible manifestation of the pain.

17.3.9 Work and benefits advice

During severe bouts of pain, patients, especially those who have personal contact with others, cannot do their jobs and so risk losing their employment. Often, after going into remission, they could go back to work but not all employers understand the unpredictability of the condition.

Box 17.1 Coping with flare-ups

- Eat mushy foods—not just potatoes and rice pudding, but a balanced diet.
- Drink with a straw.
- Keep a pain diary.
- If medications become ineffective or the side effects intolerable, get advice from specialists.
- Make decisions on which surgery to opt for when in remission, not when in severe pain.
- Vitamin B12 may be of benefit.
- Avoid going to emergency rooms unless the pain attacks are really prolonged (over 30 minutes).
- Use local anaesthetic as a spray or ointment at the site of the pain, or ask the dentist for a lidocaine injection if the pain is in the mouth.
- Contact a specialist in the case of malnutrition or dehydration as a hospital admission may be necessary.

17.3.10 'Taboo' subjects

Patients feel embarrassed about discussing some issues with their HCP. Queries can range from 'How much of my hair will be shaved off for the microvascular decompression procedure?' to lengthy discussions about personal hygiene, the loss of physical intimacy with a partner due to the fear of touching the face, hugging and kissing, or their sex lives. Mental health issues can arise, including feeling suicidal.

17.4 Benefits of support groups

Benefits of support groups include:

- Education of both patients and HCPs.
- Sense of belonging, decreasing the isolation.
- Opportunities to meet people who really understand—buddy system.
- Exchange of advice, often very practical.
- Alerting patients to research projects.
- Providing input for public and patient involvement in research projects.

17.5 Help offered by support groups

Help is provided in a number of ways. The varied activities support groups can provide are shown in fig. 17.4.

17.5.1 Helplines: support and interaction through telephone and email

Support groups provide individual support for members through email and dedicated telephone helplines that are available 24 hours a day. Volunteers are selected based on their experience and commitment, often being TN patients themselves or carers. They receive initial comprehensive instruction and ongoing development training as well as support.

Support group leaders would never seek to diagnose a caller, but their personal experience, in-house training, and accumulated knowledge gives them the ability to make suggestions or guidance towards other resources.

Support groups advise patients how to prepare for consultations, for example, keeping a pain diary and preparing their TN history, including past and present medications and side effects. They will have the information needed to advise and guide the caller to specialist teams.

In an average year in the UK, with a membership of around 1300, up to 600 calls may be dealt with and 300 email requests answered.

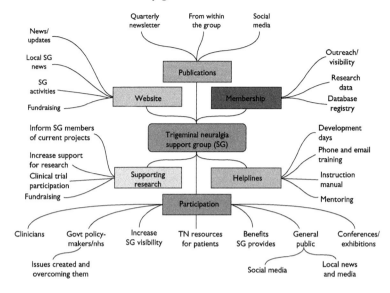

Figure 17.4 Support groups and what they can offer to patients and healthcare professionals in diagnosis and management of patients with TN

This may vary from country to country.

17.5.2 Online forum: community, validation and self-empowerment

> The fellowship of those who bear the mark of pain: who are these members of this fellowship? Those who have learnt by experience what physical pain and bodily anguish mean, belong together all the world over; they are united by a secret bond.
>
> Albert Schweitzer

TNA UK created an online forum for people affected by TN. In the first 5 years of its existence (2008–2013), the forum attracted contributions amounting to over 2 million words and covering all sorts of topics, including symptoms, medication and its side effects, surgery, living with TN, and so on. Most importantly, through the forum, those with TN become part of a group that is not constrained by geographical boundaries. This is a well-known advantage of online support groups but is particularly important for people with rare conditions such as TN, who may find it difficult to meet other sufferers in their local area.

In addition to overcoming geographical boundaries, online support groups provide a unique combination of anonymity and intimacy that creates the conditions for emotional disclosure, mutual support, and validation. On the one hand, contributors can decide how much personal information they wish to provide, including, for example, whether or not to use their real names. On the other hand, this relative anonymity makes it easier to reveal intimate details about one's circumstances (both physical and mental) that may be too embarrassing to disclose in face-to-face contexts, and sometimes too upsetting to share with family and friends. As one contributor put it, 'I am really feeling sorry for myself at the moment and just came here to get it off my chest really.'

Because members are all 'in the same boat', the forum is often used to share pain experiences, in ways that are not always possible elsewhere:

> How many times during our suffering has someone asked you 'What does it feel like?' Pain is probably the worst thing to put into words, sometimes when I describe it to someone I get the 'Wish I never asked' look from them, how about we 'share' our pain descriptions?

There is an invaluable *validation process* that takes place when patients exchange their personal experiences, and common responses are: 'That's exactly how my pain feels!' and 'It's such a relief to talk to someone who truly understands.' The process is a major factor in developing a more positive outlook for the patients.

Through regular interactions and feelings of intimacy, forum contributors can therefore come to share social and personal bonds that are as strong as those they may have with the people they interact with offline. One striking linguistic feature of the forum is the different ways in which people encourage one another and express empathy and understanding. For example, the words that are used much more frequently on the forum than in general English include:

- 'Love': e.g. 'Sending lots of love and hugs to you'.
- 'Hope': e.g. 'Hope you are still pain free'.
- 'Everyone': e.g. 'I hope everyone is ok'.
- 'Sorry': e.g. 'Sorry to hear that you are suffering'.

A common response to individuals who share difficult circumstances is 'We're all here for you'.

17.5.3 Website, printed materials, and conferences

Considerable misinformation and often dangerous advice are widespread throughout the internet and on many Facebook pages. Therefore, there is tremendous value in having a registered charity such as TNA UK which provides an informative website (https://www.tna.org.uk) and printed information that has been checked by a qualified Medical Advisory Board. Support group websites are useful sources of information for employers, and most TN associations provide excellent publications and factsheets on disability aids and benefits advice for those unable to continue working.

Support groups send out newsletters quarterly or monthly, both in hard copy and electronically. They contain information from the chairperson of the organization, current research developments, updates on upcoming events, other activities, and fundraising news.

Conferences include talks by specialists, which are greatly appreciated. Carers and family members find greater understanding and empathy by sharing with others in the group. Recent conferences have included HCPs as joint participants, and evaluations have shown how much both groups learn from these encounters. The information acquired can often correct long-held misconceptions and myths among HCPs as well as patients. Some examples of what support groups do are shown in fig. 17.5.

17.5.4 Local support groups

Not all patients can travel to a national conference so local support groups are another way of patients being able to meet. With increasing skills acquired in using internet platforms for communications, meetings through online platforms such as Zoom may be another way of involving more members.

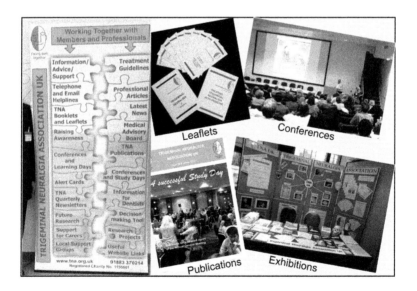

Figure 17.5 Examples of ways in which TNA UK provides support

17.6 RECOMMENDED READING

Brown JA, Ciemnecki A, editors. Facial Pain: A 21st Century Guide: For People with Trigeminal Neuropathic Pain. Los Angeles, CA: Facial Pain Association; 2020.

Zakrzewska JM. Insights: Facts and Stories Behind Trigeminal Neuralgia. Gainesville, FL: Trigeminal Neuralgia Association; 2006.

Zakrzewska JM, Jorns TP, Spatz A. Patient led conferences—who attends, are their expectations met and do they vary in three different countries? Eur J Pain. 2009;13:486–91. doi: 10.1016/j.ejpain.2008.06.001

Websites

Australia: https://www.tnaaustralia.org.au/

Canada: https://sites.google.com/view/catna/home

UK: https://www.tna.org.uk/, cluster headache https://ouchuk.org/

UK: TN: https://www.tna.org.uk/ Cluster Headache: https://www.ouchuk.org (organisation to support patients with cluster headaches and associated conditions.

USA: https://fpa-support.org, can download booklet FPA patient guide 2020.

17.7 Continuing professional development

1. What are the key objectives of patient support groups?
2. An academic linguist analysed a patient support group forum. List four key findings.
3. What can a support group provide for its members?

CHAPTER 18

Challenges and opportunities

Joanna M. Zakrzewska, William P. Cheshire Jr, and Turo Nurmikko

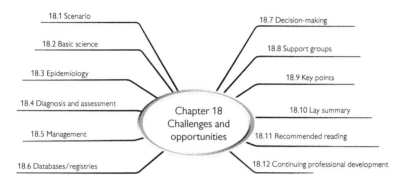

18.1 Scenario

18.2 Basic science

18.3 Epidemiology

18.4 Diagnosis and assessment

18.5 Management

18.6 Databases/registries

Chapter 18
Challenges and
opportunities

18.7 Decision-making

18.8 Support groups

18.9 Key points

18.10 Lay summary

18.11 Recommended reading

18.12 Continuing professional development

Figure 18.1 Plan of chapter

18.1 KEY POINTS

1. Several open questions remain regarding the pathophysiology of trigeminal neuralgia (TN) and other cranial neuralgias that require more research.
2. Several *in vitro* and *in vivo* assays of the trigeminal nerve are available but have not been utilized for this research.
3. Human genetic studies have discovered several candidate genes for familial TN.
4. Neuroimaging shows substantial potential.
5. More large, controlled trials with long follow-up are needed to evaluate the efficacy of pharmacological and surgical interventions in all conditions. Outcome measures require more validation.
6. Disease-specific registries held by multiple centres are recommended.
7. Patient decision-making and support group functions require more study.

18.2 Introduction

18.2.1 Scenario

A patient support charity has received a large bequest from a will with the express condition of using it for research. What would you use it for?

There are many areas where research needs to be done in order to improve outcomes for patients with trigeminal neuralgia (TN) and other nerve-mediated painful conditions of the head as shown in fig. 18.2.

Up until recently there has been relatively little research specifically on cranial neuralgias. One of the challenges of clinical practice is finding ways around the maze of uncertainties that complicate the management of these conditions. They erode our understanding of aetiology, pathophysiology, clinical features, use of investigations, choice of treatment, and prognostics. In this chapter we present some of these challenges as research questions. We also suggest a range of options that are available or can be developed to answer these research questions. They offer opportunities that medical advances have generated and can be realized using today's methodologies. While our focus is on TN, the same research need is relevant to other cranial neuralgias and trigeminal autonomic cephalalgias (TACs).

18.3 Basic science

There are several gaps in our knowledge of functional neuroanatomy, physiology and pathophysiology, neurochemistry, immunology, neuropharmacology, and surgery, raising several questions that need addressing:

- Can we establish the site and cellular and molecular mechanisms that define pain generators, for both paroxysmal pain and continuous pain (and the longer-lasting pain, e.g. in cluster headache)?

- More specifically, what intra- and extracellular mechanisms can be delineated at pain generator sites? For example, expression of which ion channels (and their subtypes) are linked to the development and maintenance of neural excitability in TN (e.g. Nav1.5, Nav1.6, Nav1.7, Cav3.2.)? Do inflammatory mediators play a role? Which neural populations are involved? Is there evidence of phenotype switching that could explain trigger zones in TN, or central sensitization that would explain one or more types of pain?

- Is there a contribution from neuroimmune communication involving glia and microglia at the ganglion level or in the central nervous system?

- Can epigenetic modifications (affecting the activity of genes encoding ion channels, neurotransmitters, and neuromodulators) be linked to alterations in the pain profiles over time?

- What is the association between genetic variants found in patients and what causes TN (and other similar conditions) and variability of phenotypes? For example, is susceptibility to neurovascular compression-induced TN or SUNCT genetically determined? Could genetic variants explain altered neural pathology sufficient to make trigeminal afferent pathways spontaneously active in TN and short-lasting unilateral neuralgiform headache

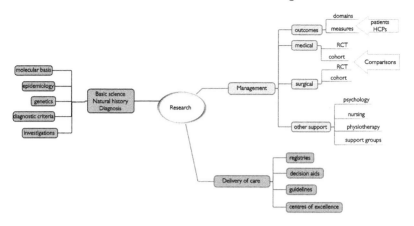

Figure 18.2 Research areas

with conjunctival injection and tearing (SUNCT), or posterior and para-
ventricular hypothalamic regions in cluster headache?

- Does descending modulation (facilitatory or inhibitory) have a role in the
pathophysiology in any neuralgia/neuropathy/TAC?

- Why do medications such as carbamazepine eventually lose efficacy following initial complete relief of pain? What are the factors that determine
the eventual return of pain following its relief by surgical procedures? For
example, can these be tracked down to altered receptor sensitivity or
epigenetic changes?

- What is the pathophysiological basis for anaesthesia dolorosa following
ablative procedures on the trigeminal nerve? For example, trigeminal
nerve cell death and compensatory hyperactivity in remaining fibres or
amplification of central signalling from increased activity in second-order
neurons or dysfunctional descending modulation?

What opportunities are there for answering any of these questions? There is no
animal model for TN but arguably some models for painful trigeminal neuropathy
and TACs. Preclinical models that are suitable for studying pain signalling in the
trigeminal system are many, and in principle can be exploited in cranial neuralgia
research although this work has not yet started. Actions of a multitude of signal
molecules can be investigated in cultured trigeminal ganglion cells. Methods to
study communication between trigeminal ganglion cells and satellite glial cells are
well developed and when put to use should provide important insights into different types of trigeminal nerve-mediated pain. Nano- and micrographic techniques allow evaluation of membrane potentials on an individual cell level. For

larger assemblies, implantable microarrays comprising over 100 microelectrodes can be used to record cortical activity in freely moving animals. In human pain studies, certain epigenetic modifications have been linked to the quality of chronic pain. Genetic studies using candidate gene approaches have identified *de novo* mutations of sodium channel Nav1.6 and whole-exome sequencing has identified rare variants in gamma-aminobutyric acid signalling and other transport genes in familial TN. Attempts are underway to engineer a TN animal model with this human mutation.

18.4 Epidemiology

Despite several studies looking at the incidence and prevalence of TN, there is no clear answer that can be used to inform service provision. One reason is less than optimal use of databases, different methods for disease classification, and data collection.

The following are some questions that need answering:

- Is there a specific geographical, ethnical distribution that may provide a clue about causality?
- What is the natural history of the condition and what are the predictors for progression?
- What are the risk factors (e.g. age, sex/gender, dental treatment, trauma to the head or mouth, elevated blood pressure, infections, diet, vitamin B12, weather, radiation, skull shape, psychological factors)?
- What is the cost of this condition to the individual and to society as a whole?

Opportunities to find answers have improved since the harmonization of classification of craniofacial pain across the three main systems (ICHD-3, ICOP, ICD-11). In them aetiological and phenotype subtypes are coded, and are easily extracted from datasets.

Analysis of large databases held by national healthcare systems such as those held by the UK NHS clinical practice research datalink (CPRD), insurance companies, regulatory agencies, or other organizations in control of population-based material will likely provide some answers.

18.5 Diagnosis and assessment

Throughout this book, one comment is constantly repeated: the diagnosis of craniofacial pain, whether TN, TAC, or other, is clinical. Lack of diagnostic biomarkers means that what really equates with a diagnosis of a given pain condition is the history and examination obtained from the sufferer, and this can only be achieved with a high level of standardization. Use of investigations whether for aetiological or pathophysiological purposes, or to predict treatment outcome, need to be robust, reliable, and repeatable, a target that has not yet been fully met. The following are some questions that need answering:

- How are the diagnostic criteria embedded in the classifications of craniofacial pain conditions validated? What are the roles of investigations in establishing precision diagnoses?
- What would a robust algorithm look like that would improve reliability of differential diagnosis of craniofacial pain conditions?
- What is the importance of the different characteristics of the pain not only in clinical differential diagnostics but also in guiding the clinicians in their treatment choices (e.g. burning vs shooting pain, or paroxysmal vs continuous pain)?
- What, if any, is the relationship of TN to the TACs?
- How do cultural, social, and psychological factors affect pain experience?
- Can objective measures of neural activity (e.g. quantitative sensory testing and laser-evoked potentials, electroencephalography, and structural or functional magnetic resonance imaging) be used (1) as a biomarker and (2) to phenotype individuals to guide personalized treatment?

Since the beginning of the millennium a great deal of work has been done in an attempt to find an answer to these questions. The ICHD-3 has undergone extensive field testing which continues. This has led to new diagnostic criteria, in particular for TN. However, more validation is needed, in particular for temporal aspects of the pain. Algorithms would be useful for training purposes and also in clinical work, and are easy to develop but so far none have been validated (see Chapter 5). Recent research has questioned the association of neurovascular coupling as the source of pain in TACs and pointed to neuronal mechanisms as the source of pain. Ongoing research is expected to show which pathophysiological features in TACs explain their clinical manifestations that differ from TN.

So far there are no validated biomarkers for any pain condition. However, there are ample opportunities for phenotyping which can be based either on characterization of pain or neurophysiological testing or neuroimaging. At present, the evidence of their usefulness comes from group studies but all are well suited for future studies on their use at individual level. These include quantitative sensory testing, laser-evoked potentials, and diffusor tensor imaging to study the microstructural changes in the trigeminal nerve and its intrapontine pathways (see Chapter 5), and functional magnetic resonance imaging to explore changes in connectivities within pain processing brain circuits.

18.6 Management

There remain very few randomized controlled trials of any form of therapy and few truly prospective longitudinal cohort studies. Thus, the challenge currently remains that the evidence base for management is poor and has been a major challenge when writing guidelines. As our understanding of the mechanisms of pain in TN, painful trigeminal neuropathy, and TACs improves, therapeutic research will be targeted requiring fewer participants with lower costs. The following are some questions that need addressing in future trials:

- What outcomes are important to patients and healthcare professionals (HCPs), and are there suitable psychometric measures available?
- What is the effectiveness and tolerability of selective sodium channel blockers such as vixotrigine, or calcium or potassium channel blockers?
- Which novel drug classes or drug development strategies show real potential (for TN, as well as other neuralgias, neuropathies and TACs, e.g. chemogenetically derived drugs, glial modulators, and drugs targeting epigenetic mechanisms)?
- How is it best to manage acute severe flare-up?
- How does provision of a cognitive behaviour programme influence outcomes?
- How do outcomes compare between medically and surgically treated patients?
- What is the most appropriate time in the course of TN to intervene surgically?
- Is neuromodulation (either non-invasive or invasive) a viable alternative for TN and painful trigeminal neuropathy (e.g. trigeminal ganglion stimulation, peripheral field simulation, epicutaneous supra-infraorbital nerve stimulation), especially in light of success of neuromodulation for cluster headache and occipital neuralgia?

Many of these challenges are being met but more work is needed. Standardization of patient-reported outcomes according to IMMPACT recommendations is being facilitated by their large-scale adoption in clinical trials. Validation is still needed for those outcomes that have been adjusted for the pain intervention in question (drugs, surgery, neuromodulation) but need more validation. Electronic diaries connected to the internet will provide real-time data collection and are becoming more sophisticated.

There are many opportunities for discoveries of novel pharmacological treatment, thanks to active preclinical pharmacological research ongoing in leading laboratories worldwide (see earlier in chapter). However, relatively few are at a stage where pivotal clinical trials could start. Several neuromodulation techniques have been trialled for TACs with promising results and technical development is continuing. The greatest advances are anticipated in non-invasive stimulation methods.

Efficacy and effectiveness studies, whether pharmacological or surgical, demand large trials and long follow-up. Recruitment into clinical trials requires collaboration of several large units with high patient turnover and suitable facilities. Participating units are likely to be centres of excellence housing a clinical trials unit with a track record of large trial output volumes.

At present, comprehensive care is available in units which are multidisciplinary and offer a full range of treatments, both medical and surgical (fig. 18.3). It is generally agreed that support should be provided by other pain HCPs such as nurses, psychologists, and physiotherapists. Self-management needs to be encouraged, and help can be provided by patient support groups. The many psychological and social consequences of chronic facial pain cannot be belittled. Suicide remains a risk factor and is highest in this group of orofacial pain sufferers. It is important to optimize data collection—patients could be encouraged to use a recording application to help them personalize their care and improve effectiveness of medications.

Fig. 18.3 shows a care pathway used in one centre in the UK.

With slight modification this care pathway can be adopted for other pain conditions as well. Equally important for the development of these types of pathways is to estimate the economic costs of the different therapies both for the individual and for the service provider.

One way forward is the setting up of national and international longitudinal cohort studies and from these identifying patients suitable for studies and comparing their outcomes to those following a different pathway as shown in fig. 18.4. Trials within cohorts encourage the use of the same core outcomes for all. Patients who would be suitable for a particular study can be randomized into those who are entered into the trial and others who are not offered the option. Those who are randomized but do not wish to take part or drop out are still followed up and can be compared to the cohort taking part as shown in a schematic presentation of a provisional trial of TN (fig. 18.4).

Large national and international studies would provide details not just on effectiveness and tolerability, but also would enable subanalysis by factors such as age, sex/gender, duration, and phenotype. Patient stratification on the basis of sensory phenotyping (using quantitative sensory testing) or neuroanatomy (small diameter nerve fibre density measured from skin biopsies) is approved for clinical trials by the European Medicines Agency, but other tests such as confocal microscopy and neuroimaging (especially diffusor tensor imaging and tractography) are easy to incorporate as entry and outcome criteria in clinical trials. All proposed trial protocols should be registered (e.g. https://www.clinicaltrials.gov/) to avoid duplication, improve recruitment and retention, and provide a site for reporting of the results.

18.7 Registries/databases

One method of improving care for patients is to set up registries that are used at multiple sites. These not only collect data from HCPs but also from patients

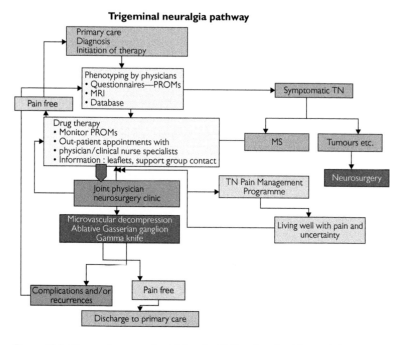

Figure 18.3 Care pathway used at University College London Hospitals for patients with TN

MRI, magnetic resonance imaging; MS, multiple sclerosis; PROMs, patient-reported outcome measures.

and are fully integrated and responsive to change. A systematic review has shown that there have been no studies of their use in the pain field, but in other areas of healthcare they have shown improved quality of care and outcomes. A registry will facilitate systematic comparison of patient populations and outcomes across multiple sites, identification of targets for improvement, and accumulation of

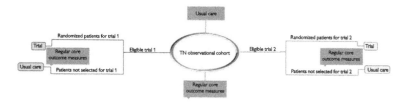

Figure 18.4 Trials within cohorts

observational data to answer research questions which cannot be answered by randomized controlled trials.

When registries are set up, some of the issues that need to be addressed include:

* Ensuring proper ethical review processes.
* Method of capture of electronic data made easy while being General Data Protection Regulation (GDPR) compliant.
* Entry criteria agreed to characterize patient population of interest.
* Centralized data completion with personnel capable of handling 'Big Data'.
* Establishing an audit process that assesses data accuracy.
* Ensuring that appropriate and transparent reporting is in place.

18.8 Decision-making

Due to the wide range of treatment options and variable outcomes, patients need help with making decisions. However, questions remain how to best achieve this aim:

* What types of aids can be developed to describe the risk of complications after surgery, and how can their validity be tested?
* How do culture, age, sex/gender, and education affect the perception of risk?
* What are the effects of shared decision-making on patient outcomes, in terms of both satisfaction and quality of life?
* Are healthcare costs reduced in patients who have high activation levels?
* Are HCPs committed to implementing shared decision-making and self-management support?

What solutions are there? There are a large number of decision aids, some of which are specific to a particular disease, whereas others are generic. One such aid is the Ottawa decision aid (https://decisionaid.ohri.ca/index.html), which can be used in combination with a consultation with an HCP. To enable determination of the usefulness of such an approach, a Patient Activation Measure (PAM) has been developed in the USA and validated in many countries including the UK. Patient activation describes 'the knowledge, skills and confidence a person has in managing their own health and health care'. Hibbard and Gilbert show that patients with high PAMs are more likely to adopt healthier behaviours and so lead to better clinical outcomes, lowered costs, and improved satisfaction. HCPs can be trained to be more effective at providing explanations that are valid, understood by patients, and action driven.

18.9 Role of support groups

Increasingly, patients will seek further advice and support outside of their HCP, and this has led to a large number of patient support groups. However, there has been little research on their impact.

The following are some questions that need to be addressed in future studies:

- How do the objectives of support groups match up with the needs and experiences of their users?
- Support groups now make full use of the internet. How does the information they provide compare to that on other social media sites, especially those that do not adhere to GDPR and quality guidelines?
- Have the support groups had an impact on HCPs and, if so, in what way?
- Do activities of the support groups reduce the use of healthcare services by sufferers and increase self-management?

18.10 Lay summary

There are numerous open questions regarding TN and other cranial neuralgias, and they range from mechanisms and type of pain and optimal treatment for each condition to the best ways to measure treatment effectiveness. Research on mechanisms and drug discovery can be conducted in the laboratory although is limited. Novel brain imaging methods and genetic tests are showing promise in identifying subgroups of people with TN. Large patient registries and support groups would help in improving patient care and help recruitment into clinical trials.

18.11 RECOMMENDED READING

Hubbard JG, Gilburt H. Supporting People to Manage their Health: An Introduction to Patient Activation. London: The Kings Fund; 2014. https://www.kingsfund.org.uk/sites/default/files/field/field_publication_file/supporting-people-manage-health-patient-activation-may14.pdf

Hoque DME, Kumari V, Hoque M, et al. Impact of clinical registries on quality of patient care and clinical outcomes: a systematic review. PLoS One. 2017;12:e0183667. doi: 10.1371/journal.pone.0183667

Nelson EC, Dixon-Woods M, Batalden PB, et al. Patient focused registries can improve health, care, and science. BMJ. 2016;354:i3319. doi: 10.1136/bmj.i3319

Petrosky E, Harpaz R, Fowler KA, et al. Chronic pain among suicide decedents, 2003 to 2014: findings from the national violent death reporting system. Ann Intern Med. 2018;169:448–55. doi: 10.7326/m18-0830

Zakrzewska JM, Relton C. Future directions for surgical trial designs in trigeminal neuralgia. Neurosurg Clin N Am. 2016;27:353–63. doi: S1042-3680(16)00023-1 [pii];10.1016/j.nec.2016.02.011 [doi]

18.12 Continuing professional development

1. How can diagnosis of the various cranial neuralgia be improved in the future?
2. What type of treatments are being put forward for possible use in TN and cranial neuralgias?
3. Why are multicentre databases/registries important?
4. How can we improve precision-based care?

Face2face: Visual journeys through trigeminal neuralgia

Ann Eastman, Alison Glenn, and Deborah Padfield

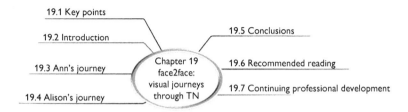

Figure 19.1 Plan of chapter

19.1 KEY POINTS

1. This project led to the creation of 54 pain cards which can be used in consultations with other patients.
2. Two patients describe their sufferings with trigeminal neuralgia, incorporating visual images they co-created.
3. The images evoke the physical pain of trigeminal neuralgia, its impact on their daily lives, and the emotional effects such as fear, low mood, and isolation.
4. Images, and the arts more widely, can be useful tools for facilitating improved interaction between healthcare professionals and patients.

19.2 Introduction

> Compassion is to look beyond your own pain, to see the pain of others.
>
> Yasmin Mogahed, 2016

While the pain of others demands compassion, it is difficult to both see and hear. It remains stubbornly resistant to language, creating a chasm between those experiencing and those witnessing it. The Face2face project at University College

London Hospital (UCLH) set out to explore whether images could be one way of negotiating this divide, making the hidden subjective experiences of pain visible and sharable through the photographic surface. Face2face was a collaboration between a facial pain consultant (Joanna Zakrzewska), an artist (Deborah Padfield), and patients and staff from UCLH NHS Foundation Trust. It explored whether photographs of pain co-created by Deborah Padfield with patients living with facial pain could facilitate improved understanding and interaction between pain patients and their treating clinicians. It asked whether such images could reinvigorate and expand the language that happens around pain in the clinic and provide an opportunity for patients to direct the consultation towards what really matters to them. Deborah Padfield worked individually with volunteers on the facial pain management waiting lists at UCLH to co-create images which reflected their unique experiences of pain. A selection of these images were subsequently integrated with photographs from a previous project at St Thomas' Hospital, 'Perceptions of pain', to form a pack of 54 laminated images or 'pain cards'. These cards were piloted in the clinics of ten experts from UCLH. The impact of the images on pain consultations has been analysed by a multidisciplinary team. This chapter presents the visual journeys of two of the core Face2face participants highlighting the intense and bewildering nature of trigeminal neuralgia pain, the fear and isolation accompanying it, and their courage and lengthy search for diagnosis and treatment.

19.3 Ann Eastman's experience

During my all-consuming career as a graphic designer, writer, and film-maker constantly travelling, plus family responsibilities, there was no time for illness. At 68 I semi-retired to freelance and 'smell the roses'.

Retired men are often struck down with heart attacks while playing golf. I was struck down by trigeminal neuralgia while brushing my teeth.

That first spasm of facial pain is unforgettable—unbearable electric shocks hammer-drilling my brain (fig. 19.2). A&E dismissed me with codeine, my puzzled general practitioner (GP) recommended ibuprofen. My dentist, perplexed by the agony emanating from a healthy tooth, regretfully extracted it. But afterwards the pain was still there!

I Googled 'phantom tooth pain' and found 'trigeminal neuralgia': the description fitted. My GP demurred; during her 40 years of experience she'd never encountered it and prescribed tramadol, temazepam, even morphine. But analgesics are ineffective for trigeminal neuralgia.

Nightmares disturbed sleep with struggles to keep doors closed against paroxysms of pain. Smiling, eating, drinking, cleaning teeth or face, or being kissed triggered episodic explosions of torture. Holidays were cancelled, theatre tickets given away, invitations declined (fig. 19.3).

Suddenly the pain vanished.

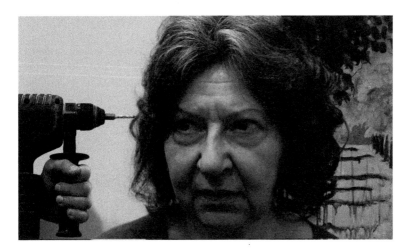

Figure 19.2 Deborah Padfield with Ann Eastman, 'Untitled' from the series Face2face, 2008–2013. Digital Archival Print

The pain of trigeminal neuralgia is beyond words. The visceral image of the hammer drill is a visual metaphor that expresses the pain.

© Deborah Padfield.

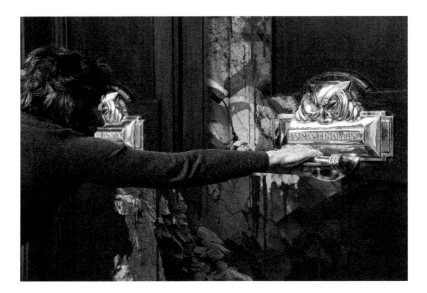

Figure 19.3 Deborah Padfield with Ann Eastman, 'Untitled' from the series Face2face, 2008–2013. Digital Archival Print

Ann's name is on the door handles. Owls were Greek symbols of wisdom, but to Celts they were evil omens. Wisdom about trigeminal neuralgia and the evil nightmare of it were behind those doors.

© Deborah Padfield.

Ten months later it returned; hammer-drilling an exploding tangle of live wires (fig. 19.4). Another tooth was extracted.

Eventually diagnosis confirmed trigeminal neuralgia. Anticonvulsants reduced the intensity of the shocks, but took four hellish weeks to achieve effectiveness.

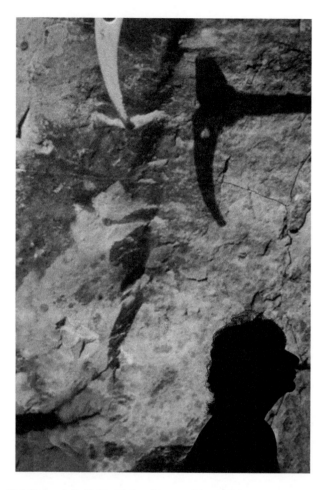

Figure 19.4 Deborah Padfield with Ann Eastman, 'Untitled' from the series Face2face, 2008–2013. Digital Archival Print

Like the Sword of Damocles—one never knows when periods of remission will end. Normal life goes on hold, creating loneliness and isolation.

© Deborah Padfield.

CHAPTER 19

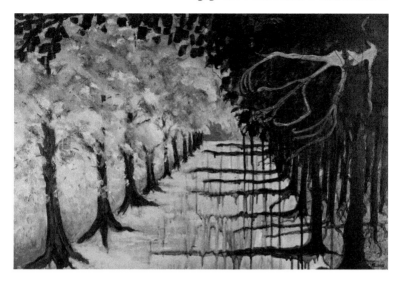

Figure 19.5 From the exhibition Mask:Mirror:Membrane, at the Menier Gallery, London, 2011
© Ann Eastman.

One's isolated life went on hold until periods of remission, but then the menace of the cosmic sledgehammer hung overhead, waiting for the next inevitable attack, but when? Possibly 2, 3, 6 months, a year ...

Collaborating in a project to create visual metaphors for diagnostic pain cards, I painted an allegorical self-portrait. The unaffected side green and bright, the afflicted side dark and bare, the trigeminal nerve's claw-like branches destroying my root structure (fig. 19.5).

Six years later, the condition escalated, striking evermore ferociously and frequently. That coincided with having to discontinue my medication, due to a potentially fatal side effect: hyponatraemia. The only remaining option was terrifying neurosurgery. According to Henry Marsh: 'All doctors have failures; the problem with brain surgery is that failure is often very terrible and very spectacular.'

Fortunately, the surgery was successful. The roses smell gorgeous (fig. 19.6).

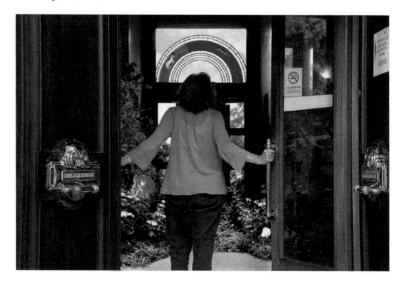

Figure 19.6 Deborah Padfield with Ann Eastman, 'Untitled' from the series Face2face, 2008–2013. Digital Archival Print

Each period of remission is like entering a paradise garden. Diagnosis and eventually surgery, if successful, makes one appreciate life.

© Deborah Padfield.

19.4 Alison Glenn's experience

My pain arrived without warning; sharp and stabbing it flashed across my jaw and although it disappeared quickly, this was the start of what became the most horrendous period in my life with recurring episodes of excruciating facial pain becoming ever more frequent and completely debilitating (fig. 19.7). Unfortunately getting a diagnosis wasn't easy. I had consultations with my GP and dentist who carried out procedures on teeth that he felt could be causing the problem. It was difficult to pinpoint exactly where the pain was as sometimes it was a sharp stabbing pain in my cheek or jaw and other times the pain came from individual teeth. Episodes of pain became very much worse after dental treatment to the point where I had difficulty even opening my mouth. I couldn't talk or eat and cleaning my teeth was an impossibility (fig. 19.8). I became very low, isolated, and unable to socialize due to the unpredictable attacks of pain.

The pain was very difficult to control and although the medication carbamazepine did give some relief, it was challenging to reach a balance between controlling the pain and being able to function normally (fig. 19.9).

After a vast number of consultations and several unnecessary root canals, I was eventually referred to the professor of facial pain, Professor Joanna Zakrzewska,

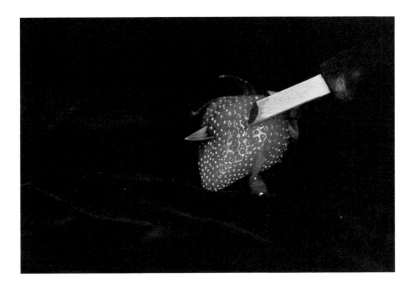

Figure 19.7 Deborah Padfield with Alison Glenn, 'Untitled' from the series Face2face, 2008–2013. Digital Archival Print

The black velvet background represents the darkness of the facial pain. The sole focus is the pain of the knife cutting through the flesh, reflected in the use of the strawberry as the focal point of the piece. The juice trickling down the strawberry conveys the idea that the pain radiates beyond the knife point.

© Deborah Padfield.

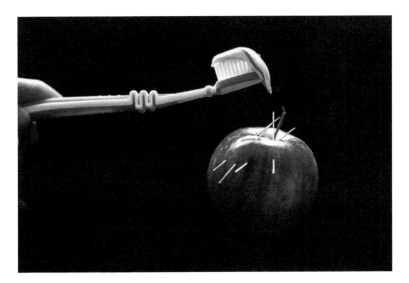

Figure 19.8 Deborah Padfield with Alison Glenn, 'Untitled' from the series Face2face, 2008–2013. Digital Archival Print

The apple was used as a reminder of the pain experienced during everyday tasks such as cleaning my teeth or eating. Despite the apple appearing to be crisp, shiny, and appetizing, it was filled with needles to represent the pain I knew that would strike if I dared to take a bite. Likewise, the toothbrush also represented a simple everyday task that I struggled to complete. The toothbrush is ready to be used, yet is untouched, just like the apple due to the daunting nature of this task.

© Deborah Padfield.

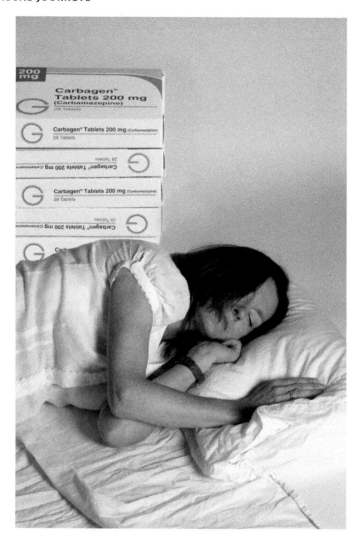

Figure 19.9 Deborah Padfield with Alison Glenn, 'Untitled' from the series Face2face, 2008–2013. Digital Archival Print

Life revolved around being reliant on medication and fearful of being without any to hand with the challenge of managing the pain while still being able to function normally.

© Deborah Padfield.

CHAPTER 19

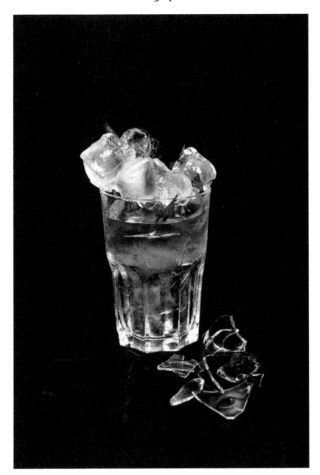

Figure 19.10 Deborah Padfield with Alison Glenn, 'Untitled' from the series Face2face, 2008–2013. Digital Archival Print

Ice cold water with hidden knife blades among the chunks of ice waiting to catch you unaware when least expected, with a sharp, stabbing cutting pain. The eye looking out from the broken glass illustrates the person experiencing the facial pain, trapped in the glass.

© Deborah Padfield.

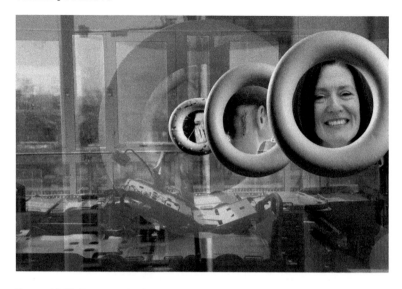

Figure 19.11 Deborah Padfield with Alison Glenn, 'Untitled' from the series Face2face, 2008–2013. Digital Archival Print

Doing this project ... was a road ... there was a beginning, middle, and end. This broke the cycle I was stuck in and I just couldn't get out of. Somehow psychologically it took me to thinking ahead, to being more positive and thinking about more positive times. It got me out of the cycle I was in.

© Deborah Padfield.

at the Eastman Dental Hospital. It took only minutes for her to diagnose trigeminal neuralgia.

Fortunately, I was a suitable candidate for surgery and although it was an incredibly invasive procedure with significant risks, I had reached a point where I couldn't cope with the pain much longer (fig. 19.10).

Thanks to the skill of a truly amazing surgeon, I have been pain free for over nine years. Being a participant on the Face2face project was a great opportunity to express and communicate my own experiences of this painful journey visually (fig. 19.11).

19.5 Conclusions

All the authors have a strong desire to promote awareness of the condition and support people with facial pain. We are keen to raise awareness among clinicians, current and future patients and carers in order to reduce suffering and the length of time before an accurate diagnosis is reached and appropriate management obtained.

19.6 RECOMMENDED READING

Ashton-James CE, Dekker PH, Addai-Davis J, et al. Can images of pain enhance patient–clinician rapport in pain consultations? Br J Pain. 2017;11:144–52. doi: 10.1177/2049463717717125

Marsh H. Do No Harm: Stories of Life, Death, and Brain Surgery. London: Weidenfeld & Nicolson; 2014. ISBN 9781780225920.

Mogahed Y. AZQuotes.com. Retrieved December 16, 2020, from AZQuotes.com website: https://www.azquotes.com/quote/1257961

Padfield D, Chadwick T, Omand H. The body as image: image as body. Lancet. 2017;389:1290–1. doi: 10.1016/s0140-6736(17)30828-0

Padfield D, Omand H, Semino E, et al. Images as catalysts for meaning-making in medical pain encounters: a multidisciplinary analysis. Med Humanit. 2018;44:74–81. doi: 10.1136/medhum-2017-011415

Padfield D, Zakrzewska JM, editors. Encountering Pain: Hearing, Seeing, Speaking. London: UCL; 2021. doi: 10.14324/111.9781787352636

Semino E, Zakrzewska JM, Williams A. Images and the dynamics of pain consultations. Lancet. 2017;389:1186–7. doi: 10.1016/S0140-6736(17)30773-0

19.7 Continuing professional development

1. How can the pain cards described in this chapter be used?
2. What were the hurdles faced by the two patients in their quest to get treatment?
3. Reflect on the impact the images in this chapter have on you.

Appendix

Answers to continuing professional development
Chapter 2
1. John Fothergill.
2. The condition was compared to epilepsy.
3. International Headache Society, International Classification of Orofacial Pain.

Chapter 3
1. Glossopharyngeal, intermedius, great auricular, and auriculotemporal nerve.
2. The site where nociceptive afferents from cranial nerves V, VI, IX, and C1–C3 converge and site of origin for ascending central pathways for these nerves. Target for descending cortical and subcortical modulation. Driver of the parasympathetic system of the head.
3. TN patients occasionally have close relatives also affected by this very rare condition, and this is consistent with their shared genes contributing to the risk of developing the condition. Recent DNA sequencing studies have found in TN patients multiple rare, damaging mutations in genes important for neuronal–glial function in the trigeminal pain network.

Chapter 4
1. Depends whether the data is from the population or from specialist centres and which criteria are used and by whom.
2. Multiple sclerosis, hypertension, strokes, depression, anxiety, and poor sleep.
3. Cluster headache.

Chapter 5
1. True: b, c, e.
2. Hereditary factors, impact on activities of daily living, carer, type of job.
3. Painful trigeminal neuropathy as there is mechanical allodynia over a larger area than just a trigger zone. On examination you are likely to also find sensory deficits to one or more modalities.

4. Beck Depression Inventory (BDI-II), Hospital Anxiety and Depression Scale (HADS), Profile of Mood States (POMS).

5. The patient has trigeminal neuralgia.

6. Social history: reflect on the impact of job loss, (mild) depression and increased catastrophizing on the patient's report of her pain and associated disability.

7. Routine MRI uses thick (3–5 mm) slices which easily miss neurovascular compression.

8. Trigeminal nerves (cisternal), root entry zone, pons at the level of intrapontine trigeminal tracts. Neurovascular compression is frequently seen at the root entry zone, multiple sclerosis plaques and isolated pontine lesions affect the central projection of the trigeminal fibres in the pons. A tumour may press the trigeminal nerve and/or pons.

9. DTI is capable of showing microstructural changes in the trigeminal pathways. The method with further development may help to understand nerve pathology when there is no significant compression, and possibly help to decide between different treatment options.

10. (i) Blink reflex, induced by stimulation of the supraorbital nerve, and the response recorded from orbicularis oris muscle. (ii) Masseter inhibitory reflex, stimulation of the mental nerve and the response recorded from the masseter muscle. Both are abnormal in patients with secondary TN.

Chapter 6

1. TN with purely paroxysmal pain and TN with concomitant (continuous) pain.

2. Yes. The classification does not rule that out. A patient with a painful trigeminal neuropathy as a complication of a neuroablative procedure for TN who goes on to experience a recurrency of TN would be diagnosed with the two concomitant conditions.

3. Unlikely. By definition, MRI will not identify either of these causes. Routine MRI is negative in temporomandibular disorders as well. The diagnosis is clinical.

Chapter 7

1. Patients with idiopathic TN do not have significant neurocompression distortion on MRI.

2. True: a, d.

3. When drug therapy is either no longer effective or poorly tolerated and quality of life has diminished.

Chapter 8

1. Two options; (1) Percutaneous neuroablative procedure, (2) MVD. Both with the warning the procedure may not be as effective as in classical TN.

2. Medical management and, if not sufficient, SRS.

Chapter 9

1. Carbamazepine and oxcarbazepine.

2. Drowsiness, dizziness, impaired cognitive function, and ataxia due to the drugs acting centrally.

3. Increase current medication or add in another one, admission would be necessary for rehydration and pain control with possible intravenous fosphenytoin.

4. Alter the drug dosage dependent on pain levels and tolerability and consider change, addition of other ones, or even stoppage during remission periods.

Chapter 10

1. MVD.

2. True: b and c.

3. Provide consultation with a neurosurgeon and physician, encourage use of a decision aid, suggest a support group, and discussion with significant others.

Chapter 11

1. ICOP-1 uses a grading system of ascending diagnostic certainty (possible, probable, definite). For the diagnosis of PTN to be considered 'definite' there has to be confirmation of trigeminal dysfunction from one or more diagnostic tests (QST, neurophysiology, skin biopsy, neuroimaging). Clinical examination including systematic sensory testing (even just using bedside tests) is necessary for meaningful clinical decision-making. A definite diagnosis is advisable before any interventional treatments. Clinical research on pathophysiology or treatment efficacy must be based on definite PTN.

2. Establish from quality and location, and clinical examination, including sensory testing of area innervated by the lingual and superior alveolar nerves (that may be injured during wisdom tooth extraction). If diagnostic uncertainty, consider neurophysiological tests and skin/mucosal biopsy and neuroimaging. Important to remember that in PTN pain may extend beyond injured nerve branch territories. Treatment of established PTN is based on pharmacotherapy, based on international guidelines, commencing with first-line drugs used for all neuropathic pain and

adding second-line drugs as necessary. Promising results are reported from use of non-invasive neuromodulation (rTMS, tDCS).

Chapter 12

1. Glossopharyngeal neuralgia, superior laryngeal neuralgia.
2. Probably combined trigeminal and glossopharyngeal neuralgia. A carefully obtained history could uncover that the pains occur independently.
3. If the patient is able and willing to undergo MVD, arrange MRI and refer to neurosurgeon. The intervention may include MVD with or without root resection, or resection alone. Non- and mini-invasive treatments (stereotactic radiosurgery, glossopharyngeal nerve radiofrequency lesioning) can be considered for those in whom posterior fossa surgery is not appropriate, but the supportive evidence is limited.
4. Stereotactic radiosurgery, possibly glossopharyngeal nerve radiofrequency ablation.

Chapter 13

1. Auriculotemporal neuralgia, greater auricular neuralgia, otic form of glossopharyngeal neuralgia, and nervus intermedius neuralgia.
2. Greater auricular neuralgia.
3. Occipital neuralgia.

Chapter 14

1. PH and HC.
2. None.
3. Vagus nerve and occipital nerve stimulation for CH.
4. SUNHA affects primarily the first division of the trigeminal nerve, which alone is rare in TN. It is associated with prominent ipsilateral autonomic features, which are rare and/or mild in TN. The number of attacks per day is much higher in SUNCT. TN patients very rarely show agitated behaviour during attacks but SUNCT patients may.

Chapter 15

1. Inflammatory conditions in the dentoalveolar complex.
2. Myofascial, temporomandibular disorders.
3. Age over 50 years, new-onset headache in temporal area, jaw claudication, visual symptoms, polymyalgia rheumatica, constitutional symptoms.
4. Burning mouth syndrome, persistent idiopathic facial pain, persistent idiopathic dentoalveolar pain.

Chapter 16

1. Depression, anxiety, fear, poor sleep, avoidance behaviour, isolation, and decrease social activities.
2. Thoughts, somatic sensations, behaviour, and emotions.
3. Statements a and c.

Chapter 17

1. Increase awareness among HCPs and public of TN and provide support to patients with TN.
2. Validation of condition, self-empowerment, increased emotional disclosure in a safe environment, allows for anonymity and intimacy, empathy.
3. Telephone, email helplines, online forums, webinars, meetings, conferences with experts, written information, advise for medical advisory board.

Chapter 18

1. Algorithms with robust screening questions, laser-evoked potentials, and neuroimaging.
2. Sodium channel blockers, chemogenetically derived drugs, and neuromodulation.
3. Epidemiological reasons, risk factors, associations, outcomes after different treatments, audit, and to improve quality of care.
4. Encourage shared decision-making, provide evidence-based information, access the impact of the condition on mood and activities of daily living so that pain management programmes can be offered, and access to support groups.

Chapter 19

1. During consultations to improve communication between patients and healthcare professionals, highlighting not only the physical aspects of pain but also the emotional and impact on activities of daily living.
2. Missed diagnosis, irreversible treatments, and significant side effects from medications.

Index

Tables, figures, and boxes are indicated by an italic *t*, *f*, and *b* following the page number.